Arthur Newsholme

School Hygiene

Or the Laws of Health in Relation to School Life

Arthur Newsholme

School Hygiene
Or the Laws of Health in Relation to School Life

ISBN/EAN: 9783337232405

Printed in Europe, USA, Canada, Australia, Japan

Cover: Foto ©Suzi / pixelio.de

More available books at **www.hansebooks.com**

SCHOOL HYGIENE:

OR

THE LAWS OF HEALTH IN RELATION TO SCHOOL LIFE.

BY

ARTHUR NEWSHOLME, M.D.,

AND DIPLOMATE IN PUBLIC HEALTH, UNIVERSITY OF LONDON; UNIVERSITY SCHOLAR AND GOLD MEDALLIST IN MEDICINE; MEDICAL OFFICER OF HEALTH FOR CLAPHAM; MEDICAL EXAMINER OF PUPIL TEACHERS TO THE SCHOOL BOARD FOR LONDON; AND MEDICAL REFEREE TO THE WESTMINSTER AND SOUTHLANDS TRAINING COLLEGES FOR TEACHERS.

BOSTON:
D. C. HEATH & CO., PUBLISHERS.
1889.

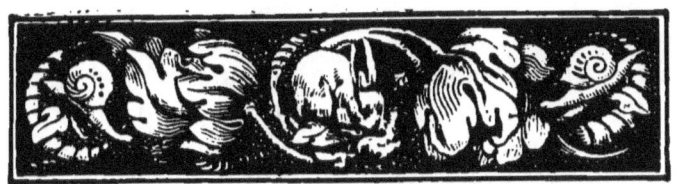

PREFACE.

THE importance of the subject here discussed must be evident to all who have bestowed even a cursory attention on the subject of popular education. As a matter of fact, it has engaged the serious attention of School Boards and Committees, and been made the subject of repeated legislation by the Education Department. The result of all this is seen in the improved character of the school-buildings which are everywhere being erected. In these, we find that greater attention is paid, not only to the space demanded for each pupil, to which a few years ago the official legislation was almost exclusively confined, but educationists have come to see that lighting, warming, ventilation, and general sanitary conditions, are of prime importance in their bearing on the health and progress of the children gathered in these schools.

Much still remains to be learnt in regard to these matters, and it is of the highest importance that school-managers and all who are concerned in the erection of school premises—or what is perhaps equally important, the modification of already existing schools—should be well acquainted with the principles which determine the sanitary condition of all school premises and arrangements.

But, however healthful the sanitary conditions of school-premises, it is evident that the health of the school must depend also largely upon the routine, the distribution of work in relation to age, the amount of exercise and rest, and other matters which concern the personal treatment of the scholars.

This branch of School Hygiene is necessarily more exclusively in the hands of the teacher, and it is therefore important that he should be well instructed in the general laws of health as applied to school-life. It is gratifying to observe that, after repeated references to the subject in their Official Reports, this has been finally recognised by the Education Department in their last Syllabus for Training Colleges, where a knowledge of the "laws of health as applied to school premises, scholars, and teachers," is made an essential part of the professional training of teachers.

The present manual has been written to supply accurate information on these two branches of School Hygiene, and it is hoped that it will be useful to all interested in the subject, and especially to those engaged in studying it in Training Colleges or elsewhere.

My own official experience as Medical Officer of Health, and as medical referee to two Training Colleges, as well as to several large private schools, has frequently forced the study of this subject upon me, and given the opportunity of becoming acquainted with its practical details. The entire subject may be regarded as a particular application of the general Laws o. Health, which I have already treated in detail in my Manual o Hygiene. The large circulation which this book has had, and its favourable reception by teachers and scientific authorities, encourage me to hope that the present work will be found equally useful and acceptable.

ARTHUR NEWSHOLME.

39, HIGH STREET,
   CLAPHAM, S.W.

CONTENTS.

PART I.—SCHOOLS.

PAGE

CHAPTER I.—SITE OF SCHOOL.

Desiderata of Site.—Level of Ground-Water.—Consumption, Rheumatism, &c., from Damp Soils.—Special Susceptibility of Children —Drainage of Soil.—Character of Soil.—School not in Main Street.—Not to be Overshadowed.—Allow for Playgrounds. 3

CHAPTER II.—CONSTRUCTION OF SCHOOL BUILDINGS.

Foundation of School.—Walls.- Style of Architecture.—Internal Wall-surfaces.—Floor.—Arrangement of Rooms.—Corridors. --Staircases.—Cloak-room.—Playground. ...

CHAPTER III.—SCHOOL FURNITURE. 7

Desks and Seats.—Evil Effects of Long-sitting in one Posture.—Varieties of Bad Desks and Seats.—Results of These.—" Distance" and " Difference."—Slope of Desk.—Height and Width of Seat.—Height of Back.—Long or Short Desk.—Desks according to Height, not Age.—Blackboard.—Pictures 12

CHAPTER IV.—LIGHTING OF SCHOOL-ROOMS.

Evil Effects of Deficient Light.—Amount of Window-area required.—Direction of Light.—Artificial Lighting ... 17

CHAPTER V.—GENERAL PRINCIPLES OF VENTILATION.

Physiology of Respiration.—Tests for Impurity of Air.—Effects of Breathing Impure Air.—Effect on Mental Powers.—Temperature of Air required.—Dryness of Air.—Amount of Air required.—Amount of Floor Space ... 21

CHAPTER VI.—NATURAL VENTILATION.

Rules Respecting Ventilation.—Natural and Artificial Ventilation.—Ventilation through Window, Wall, Chimney, Ceiling. 29

CHAPTER VII.—VENTILATION AND WARMING.

Difficulties of Successful Ventilation by Warm Air.—Open Fire-place.—Heating by Gas.—Closed Stoves.—Central System of Heating.—Hot Air Furnaces.—Steam Apparatus. —Hot Water Apparatus. -Entrance Flues and Extraction Shafts.—The Bridgeport System 36

CHAPTER VIII.—DRAINAGE ARRANGEMENTS.

Lavatories.—Urinals.—Water-closets.—Soil-pipe.—Drains.—Earth-closets 46

PART II.—SCHOLARS.

	PAGE

CHAPTER IX.—MENTAL EXERCISE.
Full Scope of Education.—Quantity and Quality of Brain.—The Brain a Compound Organ.—Functional Habits of Brain – Blood Supply.—Sensory and Muscular Education of Brain 57

CHAPTER X.—EXCESSIVE MENTAL EXERCISE.
Symptoms and Effects of Brain-forcing.—The "Cram" System.—Causes of Over-strain.—Home Lessons.—Badly-arranged Work.—Importance of Technical Instruction.—Good and Bad Examinations.—Consumption from Overwork.—Punishments 62

CHAPTER XI.—AGE AND SEX IN RELATION TO SCHOOL WORK.
Duration of School-work at various Ages.—Statistics of Children attending School at various Ages.—Growth and Development in Relation to School-work.—Weight and Size of Children.—Chart of Growth of Children.—Sex in Education.—Character of Education in Relation to Sex. 70

CHAPTER XII.—MUSCULAR EXERCISE AND RECREATION.
Analogy between Mental and Muscular Exercise.—Influence of Exercise on the System.—Influence on the Brain.—Excessive Exercise.—Deficient Exercise.—Rules for Exercise.—Forms of Exercise.—Gymnastics.—Calisthenics ... 83

CHAPTER XIII.—REST AND SLEEP.
Law of Rest and Action.—Partial Rest —Complete Rest.—Duration of Sleep.—Rules respecting Sleep.—School Dormitories 91

CHAPTER XIV.—CHILDREN'S DIET.
Quantity and Quality of Food.—Food required for Growth.—Relation of Food to Work.—Frequency of Under-feeding.—Amount of Food Required.—School Dietaries.—Water at School. 95

CHAPTER XV.—CHILDREN'S DRESS.
Amount of Clothing Required.—Relation of Clothing to Food—The Hardening Process.—Distribution of Clothing.—Rules respecting Clothing 99

CHAPTER XVI.—BATHS AND BATHING.
Necessity for Cleanliness.—School Baths and Swimming ... 102

CHAPTER XVII.—EYESIGHT IN RELATION TO SCHOOL LIFE.
Structure of the Eye.—Causation of Long and Short Sight.—Use of Eyes for Near Objects.—Inadequate Light.—Badly Printed Books.—Fine Needlework.—Influence of General Health on Eyesight. 104

Contents.

	PAGE
CHAPTER XVIII.—COMMUNICABLE DISEASES IN SCHOOLS. Moral Duty of Parents and Medical Men.—Symptoms of Onset of Infectious Diseases.—Rules for Guidance of Teachers.—Duration of Infection.—Isolation of Healthy Members of Household.—Diseases from Insanitary Schools.—Question of Closing Schools for Epidemics.—Management of Infectious Diseases in Boarding Schools.—Other Communicable Diseases.—Ringworm.—Itch.	116
CHAPTER XIX.—SCHOOL ACCIDENTS. Importance of First Aid.—Fainting.—Fits.—Suffocation.—Drowning.—Foreign Bodies.—Stings and Bites.—Wounds.—Hæmorrhage.—Nose Bleeding and Spitting of Blood.—Fractures.—Dislocations.—Sprains.—Contusions.—Concussion.—Football.	131
INDEX	141

LIST OF ILLUSTRATIONS.

FIG.		PAGE
1	Diagram of foundation and damp-proof course	8
2	Diagram of desk and seat	15
3	Ventilating gas-pendant	20
4	Ventilation by hinged window	31
5	Ventilation between window-sashes	32
6	Ventilation by Tobin's tube and exit-shaft from centre flower of ceiling	33
7	Sheringham's ventilator	33
8	Boyle's mica flap ventilator	34
9	Slow combustion ventilating-stove	38
10	The Calorigen stove	39
11	Closed stove arranged to warm incoming fresh air	41
12	Lavatory wash-basin	47
13	Pan-closet with D trap beneath	48
14	An improved valveless closet	49
15	A sanitary valve-closet	50
16	Section of disconnecting chamber for school-drain	51
17	Iron cover to disconnecting chamber	52
18	Chart of height and weight from birth to 25 years of age	79
19	Chair giving complete spinal support	87
20	Vertical section of the eyeball	105
21	Diagram showing effect of biconvex lens on rays of light	106
22	Section of hypermetropic eye	107
23	Section of myopic eye	109
24	Chart showing prevalence of near-sight and far-sight at different ages	111
25	The Itch Insect	125
26	A burrow formed by the Itch Insect in epidermis	126
27	Ringworm	128
28	The inspiratory movement in artificial respiration	133
29	The expiratory movement in artificial respiration	134

PART I.
SCHOOLS.

SCHOOL HYGIENE.

CHAPTER I.

SITE OF SCHOOL.

Desiderata of Site.—Level of Ground-Water.—Consumption, Rheumatism, &c., from damp Soils.—Special Susceptibility of Children.—Drainage of Soil.—Character of Soil.—School not in Main Street.—Not to be Overshadowed.—Allow for Playgrounds.

FREQUENTLY no choice can be exercised as to the site of a school. The school already exists, and must be adapted as best can be for its purposes. Or, again, the site is determined by arbitrary and inevitable circumstances, such as the question of expense of ground, central position for the children, &c.

In all cases where a choice is possible, the following requirements should be carefully fulfilled; and where an unsuitable site has already been occupied, it should be brought as far as possible in accord with the conditions to be named.

(1.) *The Level of the Ground or Subsoil Water* must be carefully ascertained. Every soil contains water at a certain level below its surface, the depth of which can be easily ascertained by finding the height of the water in the nearest shallow well. The basement-floor should be at least three feet above the highest level of the ground-water. A soil in which the ground-water is usually low, but liable to sudden variations in level, is less healthful than one in which the water is somewhat near the surface, but without great alternations. The close relationship of Consumption to excessive moisture of soil has been clearly demonstrated in England by Dr. Buchanan, and in America by Dr. Bowditch, of Boston.

Rheumatism, likewise, is favoured by damp and ill-drained sites.

When a damp soil contains decomposing vegetable matters, under the influence of the warmth of late summer and autumn months, malarious diseases are liable to be produced.

Ague, the type of malarious diseases, was formerly prevalent in southern New England, around New York City, and many parts of New Jersey. Improved drainage, and the consequent increased dryness of soil, have, however, almost entirely abolished it. Diphtheria, again, seems to be connected in its origin with a damp soil, though, in this case, a defective condition of sewerage is generally associated with the dampness.

In connection with all these conditions, children are much more prone to suffer than adults. Their resisting powers are smaller, and they sooner fall victims to the results of bad hygienic conditions.

(2.) *Drainage of Soil.* — No matter how dry may be the natural condition of a soil, a site without means of drainage should not be accepted at any price. Even a clay soil may be made comparatively warm and dry by means of brick or perforated earthenware pipes. These should preferably not run into any part of the sewerage system, but into the nearest water-course. If it is necessary to join them with a sewer, their contents should not pass directly into it, but into a disconnecting trap.

(3.) *Character of the Soil.*—" Made " soils, often consisting of the refuse and garbage collected from dust bins, should be carefully avoided. The gradual putrefaction of such organic matters, leads to the production of effluvia, which mount into the school-rooms, and may develope diphtheria and other diseases. Sandy, or coarse gravel soils are to be preferred. Clay soils are cold and retentive of moisture, unless very well drained.

(4.) *Relation of Site to surrounding Objects.*—The neighbourhood of stagnant pools or marshy ground is to be studiously avoided, as it is open to the dangers which are necessarily associated with the slow putrefaction of organic matters. The vicinity of any factory, or other establishment liable to poison the air with offensive effluvia, should likewise be avoided.

India-rubber works, tar.-yards, bone-boiling and soap-making establishments are particularly objectionable. The neighbourhood of gas-works is objectionable in a minor degree. If the neighbourhood of a factory or workshop is associated with the noise of machinery, serious interference with school-work may result.

Position in a main street is by no means always advisable. Apart from the noise which interferes with attention to school-work, there is more danger of children being run over while hurrying from school, than if the exit is in a side street. Proximity to foundries, railway stations, markets, or stables is undesirable. The close neighbourhood of trees, except to north or east, is to be deprecated, and then they should not be sufficiently near to impede the free entrance of light or air. The close vicinity of higher buildings is for similar reasons objectionable.

The site should be sufficiently extensive to allow for playgrounds. This is not only necessary for recreation, but it prevents to some extent the overshadowing of surrounding buildings. At least two adjoining sides of the school should be freely exposed to light and air, and at a distance of not less than 60 feet from any other building.

CHAPTER II.

CONSTRUCTION OF THE SCHOOL BUILDINGS.

Foundation of School — Walls.—Style of Architecture.—Internal Wall-surfaces.—Floor.—Arrangement of Rooms. —Corridors.— Staircases.—Cloak-room.—Playground.

IT is most convenient to discuss first the general construction and arrangement of school buildings, leaving the subjects of lighting, ventilation, warming, and drainage to later chapters.

The School Foundation requires to be solid and substantial and made as nearly as possible impervious both to moisture and air, in order to cut off the ground-air, which is otherwise drawn into heated rooms, and may contain the germs of diphtheria, enteric fever, or some other disease. Impervious concrete, hydraulic cement, asphalted brick, or sheet-lead are among the best materials for this purpose. The impervious material should reach on each side at least six inches beyond the frontage of the wall. (Fig. 1.)

The Walls should likewise have special arrangements for preventing the rise of damp. Two layers of roofing slate set in cement, or a layer of good asphalte, or a course of perforated glazed tiles, form a good damp-proof course. When we remember that a common brick will absorb a pint of water, and that moisture rises along the bricks of a building, just as it would run up a series of lumps of sugar arranged on the top of each other, the importance of this matter will be realised.

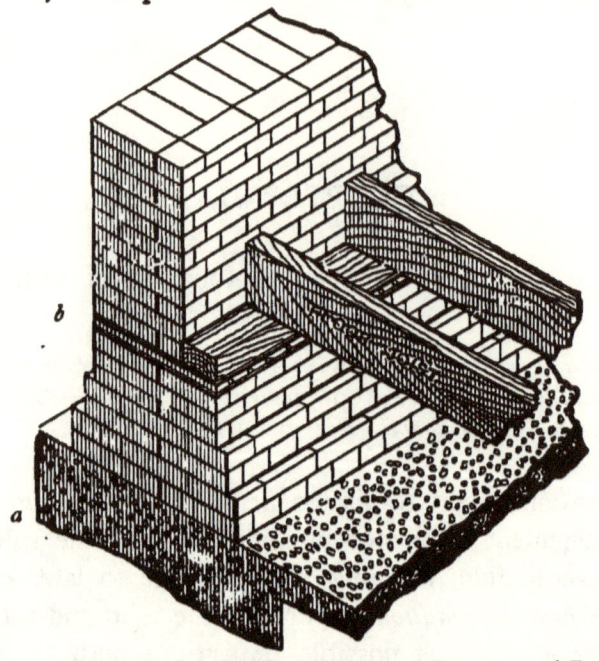

FIG. 1.—Diagram showing Foundation and Damp-proof Course.
a. Concrete Foundation. *b.* Damp-proof Course

The Style of Architecture may be regulated according to local circumstances, but should be such as not to be an offence to the eye, or out of harmony with its environment. Expensive ornamentation should never be indulged at the expense of efficient ventilating or warming apparatus.

The Internal Wall-surfaces should not be papered, as they cannot then be frequently cleansed. If simply white-washed or colour-washed, the plaster of the room for a time serves to neutralise the carbonic acid from respiration, but afterwards this action ceases, and the walls become saturated with volatile organic matters from respiration, &c., which tend to maintain the atmosphere in an impure condition, even though fresh air is admitted. Washable distempers are very good, and they present the advantage that their colouring matter does not rub off on the clothes.

It is preferable to have impervious polished walls, made thus by painting, or by polished cement, or tiles. These can be frequently washed, and thus the atmosphere kept sweet and pure If the walls are coloured, the tints should be cream or light brown, or a pale blue or green.

The wainscoting should be four to five feet high. All projections which can harbour dust should be as far as possible abolished. Thus cornices are objectionable, and the tops of doors and windows should be levelled off.

The Floor of the school-room should be constructed of narrow planks, with dovetailed or matched joints. The wood should be close-grained and hard, so as not easily to splinter. Wood floors are warmer than asphalte or brick. The floor may be washed during the school recess, but must be well dried. A better plan is to have it beeswaxed and polished at intervals: it then only requires sweeping each day.

The Floor Plan should be carefully devised. A form of building in which a central corridor is surrounded by class-rooms on three or four sides is not advisable, as it does not allow a free circulation of air. A better arrangement is to have rooms on only one side of a corridor, so that the chief light comes from one side of the rooms. The best shape for school-rooms is an oblong, the sides of which bear the proportion of about 4 to 3, each room allowing 150 cubic feet per pupil, of which at least 15 square feet should be floor-space. The minimum Government requirement in England is 80 cubic feet per pupil, not less than 8 square feet of which must be allowed for floor-space. In common lodging-houses, if the cubic space allowed per individual is below 300 cubic feet, the proprietor is liable to prosecution. We are therefore not overstating the matter in saying that 150 cubic feet per pupil is desirable in a school.

Corridors should be large, airy, and well lit. If they are cramped for space, or have not an abundance of direct light the ventilation of the school is sure to suffer.

Staircases should be fire-proof, and so situated that, in case of fire, there is easy access to them. There should be two separate flights of stairs, neither of which should be directly opposite a door. A landing should break the stairway about every 15 steps, in order to avoid falls from a great height. The door should open outward toward the street, to prevent a block in case of panic, and the doorway should always be wider than the stair which leads to it. Spiral stairs without landings and having tapered steps are most objectionable.

Cloak-rooms should be provided in every public school, the children's outer clothing and umbrellas never being allowed in the school-room. Each child should have a separate numbered place for hanging his outdoor costume. By this means the danger of wetting one another's clothes and of infection is minimised.

There should be a system of umbrella-drainage, channels communicating with all the compartments, to carry the drippings straight out of the school. A system of hot-water or hot-air pipes should run under all the compartments, so as to subject each coat, hat, and umbrella to a current of hot air and dry them. To facilitate rapid and orderly assembly and dismissal, it is desirable that there should be a separate cloak-room for each 120 to 150 scholars, contiguous to the respective class-rooms. It should be well ventilated to carry off the vapour produced by wet clothing.

The Playground should be as large as circumstances will allow. If possible, it should not be on the north or east side of the school, the south or west being preferred. A portion of it should be covered, especially in the case of infant-schools. This may be obtained by having a light shed, open at one side, or, if ground is expensive, by raising the school on a low story, eight to nine feet high, and using the ground underneath as a covered playground. Some of the recently built public schoolhouses in England have flat roofs for playground purposes. If due precautions are taken to prevent the possibility of accidents, this plan may be very serviceable where economy of space is essential.

CHAPTER III.

School Furniture.

Desks and Seats.—Evil results of long-sitting in one posture.—Varieties of bad Desks and Seats.—Effects of these.—"Distance" and "Difference."—Slope of Desk.—Height and Width of Seat.—Height of Back.—Long or Short Desk.—Desks according to Height, not Age.—Blackboard.—Pictures.

DESKS AND SEATS are the most important articles of school furniture, and it is unfortunate that authorities on this subject are not agreed as to their best form.

It is well to remember at the outset that no form of desk or seat will obviate the evils of long continuance in any one position. This leads to imperfect expansion of the lungs, relaxation of muscles, and a tendency to drooping shoulders, if not actually to a twist in the spinal column. A few moments' interval during a writing lesson, devoted to arm exercises, will be extremely beneficial in maintaining proper postures.

Various bad forms of DESK are met with. The desk may be *too high*, in which case, during writing, one shoulder is unduly raised in order to rest the arm on the desk, and a lateral twist of the spine results, which, in time, tends to become persistent. If the desk is *too low*, the scholar has to bend too far over his work. A forward stoop and round shoulders are produced; the head becomes congested from being held so low, and there is a strong tendency for the development of near-sightedness. (See Chapter XVII.)

A flat desk is particularly bad, necessitating a cramped position, and interference with free respiration.

If the *desk is too far from the seat*, a forward stoop, with round shoulders, flat chest, and injury to the eyes, is produced.

SEATS, again, may be badly placed. If the seat is *too high*, the feet swing, the vessels and nerves at the back of the legs are compressed, and the sensation of "pins and needles." is produced. This is also very apt to occur if, as is commonly the case, the seat is too narrow to support the whole length of the thigh. If *too low*, the thighs are bent up towards the body, and a cramped position is produced. If without a *back-rest*, or with an improperly adapted back-rest, the pupil tends to lean forward on the desk, and thus prevent free expansion of the lungs.

Ill Effects of bad Desks and Seats.—According to Eulenberg, a distinguished German orthopædic surgeon, 90 per cent. of curvatures of spine not caused by actual bone-disease, are developed during school life. Bad postures during school work, and especially the twisted position, with the left arm resting on the desk during writing lessons, contribute considerably to the production of such curvatures. The effects are much more likely to be produced if desk and seat are not properly adapted to each other, and to the size of the pupil. An upright position in writing is indispensable, and the left elbow should not be allowed to rest high up on the desk. Writing should be continued for only a few minutes in infant and junior classes, and in higher classes not longer than half-an-hour, without intermission.

The cramped positions induced by defective desks and seats, not only favour the production of a twisted spine, but also round shoulders and flat chest, thus impeding the functions of heart and lungs. The habit of leaning forward close over the copy-book or reading-book, may produce shortsightedness; and this in its turn increases the necessity for the improper postures. Thus a vicious circle is entered, each evil mutually intensifying the other.

Proper Desks and Seats should be accurately adapted to each other. The most important points to ascertain are the "Distance," *i.e.*, the distance between the edge of the seat and a perpendicular line dropped from the edge of the desk; the "Difference," *i.e.*, the difference between the height of seat and desk; and the slope of the desk. (Fig. 2.)

The Distance should, for writing purposes, equal zero,—the plumb line from the desk grazing the edge of the seat,—or it should be a negative quantity. For other purposes the distance should equal zero or a small positive quantity. This involves having a moveable seat, unless chairs are used, which is inadvisable in boys' schools. Or, the same end may be attained by using a desk so constructed that it can be drawn horizontally backward, so as to enable the scholar to write while sitting erect, or resting his back against the back of the seat. When the scholar is too far away from the desk, he either bends forward into an unnatural position, or glides too far forward on his seat, and occupies an unsteady position.

The *Difference* between height of seat and desk should not be such that the shoulders are painfully screwed up in writing, or, on the other hand, the pupil is obliged to lean forward in order to write or read. It is recommended that it should equal the length of the forearm, or about one-sixth the height of the scholar (Robson), in which case it will be found that the under-part of the forearm will rest comfortably on the desk-top.

The Slope of the Desk should be capable of change, the proper angle being about 30° for writing and 40°-45° for reading.

The Height of the Seat should correspond to the length of

the scholar's leg from sole of foot to knee, in order that there may be no stretching of muscles. Its *width* should not be under eight inches.

There should be a *back* to the seat, which need not be more than a piece of wood 3 inches broad, slightly tilted back, and so placed as to support the back just below the shoulder blades. In this way the movements are not interfered with, while the spine receives steady support. Liebreich gives the rule that the top of the back of the seat should be an inch lower than the edge of the desk for boys, and an inch higher than the same point for girls.

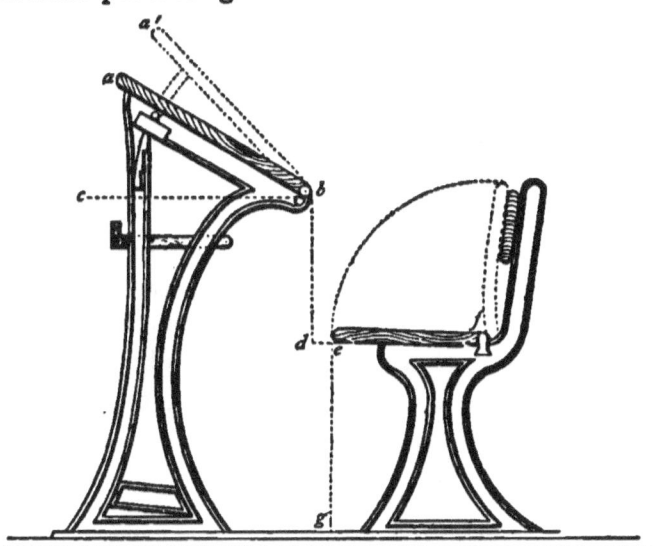

FIG. 2.--Diagram of Desk and Seat.

$a\,b\,c$, angle of 30° for writing. $a'\,b\,c$, angle of 45° for reading ; $b\,d=\frac{1}{8}$ height of scholar; $e\,f=$at least 8 inches ; $e\,g=$length of scholar's leg from knee to sole of foot ; $d\,e=$not more than 1 inch for reading, and zero for writing, and preferably zero for both. $b\,d=$" Difference." $d\,e=$" Distance."

Long desks are, as a rule, objectionable : children tend to sit with the left arm high up on the desk, in order to prevent copying by their neighbours, and thus produce twisting of their spines. The same objection holds against dual desks to a less extent, but they possess the advantage of not spreading out the children so much as single desks, and thus economise the teacher's voice. They also suffice for three, when listening to a lesson.

It is a common fault to furnish a room with desks of only one size. There should be three sizes of desks in each large class-room, as there may be great diversity of height among children differing only two or three years in age. A foot-rest should always be provided for children varying considerably from the usual stature.

Other articles of school furniture require little notice.

The Black Board should be large. It should be so placed as to receive a good light, and its surface should be dull. The windows of the school-room should not be on the same wall as the black board, as otherwise the children's eyes are dazzled in looking at the board.

Pictures in schools have a great educational value. None are so easily affected and impressed by their surroundings as children. Hence the importance of surrounding them with beauties of form and colour, thus fostering their taste, while the daily discipline of school life promotes habits of order. A common fault to be avoided is having the pictures too small.

CHAPTER IV.

Lighting of School-rooms.

Evil Effects of Deficient Light.—Amount of Window-area required.—Direction of Light.—Artificial Lighting.

THE depressing effects of a dull day, which largely depend on the absence of direct sunlight, are sufficiently known to all. Light and happiness seem necessarily associated, and are even used as synonymous in the well-known verse—" Light is sown for the righteous, and gladness for the upright in heart."

The best way to stop a canary singing is to cover his cage with a shade; and the bright spirits of children are similarly affected by dull dark school-rooms. The mental effect of deficient light is accompanied by an actual physical effect. Plants grown in the dark are weakly and white; and human beings under similar conditions become pale and comparatively bloodless (anæmic). "Where the light cannot come, the doctor must," is a proverb expressing this truth in a pithy form. The attendance in a badly-lit school is always less regular than in a cheerful well-lit school.

Small windows, often half shaded by blinds, and seldom as clean as they might be, are common defects in our schools. The furniture and paints, again, are not uncommonly daik-coloured, which increases the general gloom. Varnishing the walls greatly improves the lighting. Not only is a badly-lit room injurious in itself, but it leads to an increased use of lamps or gas, thus bringing into action another source of impurity.

The Window Area required in a school-room is variously stated as from one-fourth to one-tenth of the floor-area of the room. The plan recommended by R. Morris is to multiply the length, breadth, and height of the room together, and take the square root of this for the area of the windows.

It is evident that the amount of window-area required will vary with external conditions. Thus, in towns more should be allowed than in the country, and more in a narrow street than where there is an uninterrupted outlook. Also, more is required in the lower than the higher stories. A greater amount of light is obtainable from skylights than from vertical windows.

Windows should always reach nearly to the ceiling, as the best light comes from the highest point, and much of the cheerfulness of a school-room depends on the amount of sky which is visible. Plate glass is preferable, being thicker, and allowing less escape of heat. Double windows check cold draughts and economise heat. They may also be made to materially help natural ventilation, by allowing an upward current between them into the room. Ground glass windows prevent glare. If the access of light is barred by an opposite wall, this may be painted or white-washed, and the use of "Daylight Reflectors" is sometimes very advantageous.

South windows admit more light than any other; but if any part of the lighting is from the roofs, do not let the skylight slope to the south or west, as the heat and light will be intolerable in hot weather.

The Direction of the Light is a matter of great importance.

The worst light is that which comes from windows facing the scholars. It throws the teacher's face into the shade, and the scholars' books are similarly affected. A light from behind obliges the scholar to sit in a twisted position, in order that his book may not be in the shade. Light from both right and left throws a double set of shadows, unless the amount of illumination from one side (which ought to be the left) is much greater than from the opposite side. If this condition is fulfilled, there is no serious objection to cross-lighting, and it greatly facilitates ventilation. The best light is that which comes directly from the left, and does not necessitate any other than an erect posture in order that it may fall directly on the desk. The lower panes of windows are of comparatively little use in admitting light for study; the light comes too horizontally, and there is more danger of dazzling the eyes.

A semicircular arrangement of the seats in a room, is disadvantageous for lighting purposes. There should be a gangway near the left-hand windows, to prevent the children nearest them being in the shade.

Excess of Light is much more easily remedied than a deficiency. Inside rolling slat-blinds answer the purpose, but external venetian or other blinds are much more effectual in keeping out the heat of the sun.

Artificial Lighting is only exceptionally required in day-schools; and the corridors should be so constructed as not to require its aid.

The electric light possesses great sanitary advantages in its freedom from injurious products of combustion, and in the fact that it does not harm books and paintings.

Gas is the usual source of artificial light. As ordinarily employed, it is pernicious, because it dries the air, produces heat out of all proportion to the light, and loads the air with noxious gases. It should never be allowed in a school-room, unless contained in a cylinder which carries off the products of combustion, either directly to the external air (Fig. 3), or into the chimney-flue. It may in this way be so arranged as to form a valuable aid to ventilation.

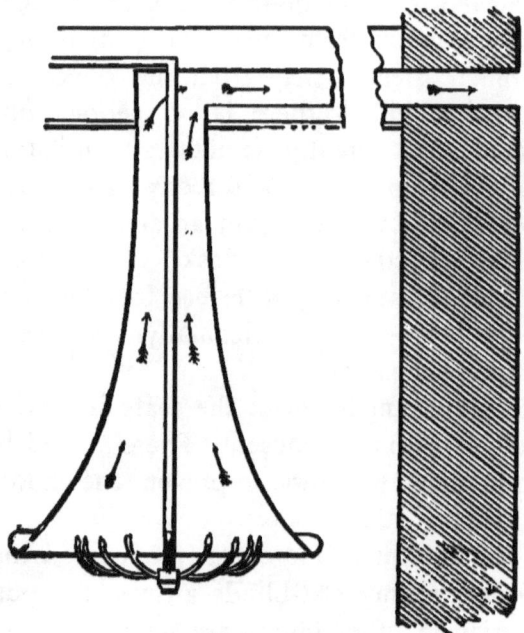

FIG. 3.—Ventilating Gas Pendant.

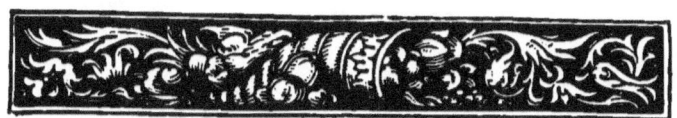

CHAPTER V.

GENERAL PRINCIPLES OF VENTILATION.

Physiology of Respiration.—Tests for Impurity of Air.—Effects of Breathing Impure Air.—Effects on Mental Powers.—Temperature of Air Required.—Dryness of Air.—Amount of Air Required.—Amount of Floor Space.

IT has been well said that "our own breath is our greatest enemy," and the problem of a healthful school-room is to a large extent solved by the application of measures for removing this, and furnishing an abundant supply of pure air, without the production of perceptible draughts.

A knowledge of the *Physiology of Respiration* is necessary before the importance of ventilation can be realised, and the amount of fresh air required can be ascertained. The essential element in the atmosphere is oxygen, a gas which is diluted by four times its volume of nitrogen, an innocent gas without any active properties. The oxygen of air is absolutely essential for the continuance of all forms of animal life. By means of our lungs, it is furnished to the system, and at the same time carbonic acid gas and other impurities are eliminated.

The windpipe carrying air down to the lungs branches repeatedly, the ultimate minute branches ending in little cavities, called air-cells, of which there are probably five or six millions, with an aggregate area of ten to twenty square feet. This large area is separated only by extremely delicate walls (so delicate as to be hardly recognisable) from the blood circulating in the lungs; and an interchange is rapidly effected, by which the blood becomes oxygenated and at the same time parts with its impurities. Now the heart is contracting from 60 to 70 times every minute, at each contraction driving the blood to every part of the body, including the lungs; and it is found that the whole blood passes through the lungs, and is subjected to this purifying influence nearly twice every minute.

The air expired differs from that inspired in several important particulars. In the first place, it has become *warmer*, having been warmed by its contact with the warm blood which is flowing through the lungs. In the next place, it is *moister*, a large amount of water-vapour being given off. By the lungs and skin conjointly, from 26 to 40 ounces of water pass off in 24 hours. Five hundred children assembled in one room would, in the course of two hours, give off as vapour about four gallons of water, which would be visible in the clouding of windows and walls, unless the room were well ventilated.

In the third place, expired air contains four per cent. less oxygen and over four per cent. more carbonic acid than that inspired. Ordinary out-door air contains four parts of carbonic acid in 10,000 of air, but in expired air this is increased to 400 parts. Healthy adults exhale about 14·4 cubic feet of carbonic acid per day. Children are said to produce less than this, but as their vital processes are more rapid than those of adults, the difference is not so great as might be expected. Five hundred children assembled in one room would in two hours produce as much carbonic acid as is equivalent to the solid charcoal or carbon contained in 20lbs of coal.

In the last place, expired air contains in suspension considerable volatile organic matter, of a highly putrefiable nature.

This is invisible under ordinary circumstances, but is none the less foul and offensive.

The carbonic acid in expired air is far from being harmless, but it is innocent as compared with these organic particles which emanate from our own bodies. When the latter are not removed by ventilation, they may be rebreathed, and thus, instead of the blood being purified twice each minute, it may be gradually vitiated and poisoned. Imagine the condition of a child who had no bath for six months; but uncleanliness of the skin is surely of less importance than of the delicate membrane lining the lungs! Besides, there is no such ready entrance into the blood from the skin as from the lungs.

If we were asked to drink foul water or eat decomposing food, we should at once refuse, but we frequently inhale air which is fouler than the dirtiest ditch-water, and nearly as offensive as a rotten egg; while our children are crowded in school-rooms in which they are forced repeatedly to breathe their own and other children's breaths, to the sad injury of their health.

Tests for Impurity of Air.—Perhaps one of the best tests for respiratory impurities, is by the sense of smell. It must be exercised, however, after a few minutes' stay in the outer air, as no sense is more quickly blunted than that of smell. On entering a room of which the atmosphere is impure, it will be found perceptibly stuffy if the carbonic acid in the air reaches 6 parts in 10,000, and the degree of stuffiness or closeness is a very fair indication of the amount of impurity present. When the amount of carbonic acid reaches 10 parts in 10,000, the room is extremely close.

A simple chemical test to ascertain if the carbonic acid amounts to 6 parts in 10,000 of air, is the following :—Procure a bottle holding $10\frac{1}{2}$ fluid ounces, blow the air of the room into it by means of a bellows, pour in half-an-ounce of lime-water, and after corking tightly, shake the bottle well for two or three minutes. If no visible milkiness is produced (by the union of carbonic acid and lime forming chalk), then the amount of carbonic acid in the room is below 6 parts in 10,000.

There is no simple test for the organic impurities in air, which are really more important, because more pernicious, than the carbonic acid; but inasmuch as the carbonic acid is nearly always in exact proportion to the amount of organic matter, the test for the former answers equally well for the latter.

This test, combined with the sense of smell on coming direct from the external air, gives most reliable indications, which should never be neglected.

Non-Respiratory Impurities of Air.—*Carbonic Oxide Gas* is produced in furnaces and stoves, and when it obtains entrance into a room, giddiness, headache, and depression of the general health are the result. Indeed, this gas is poisonous in much smaller quantities, and much more quickly than the closely-allied compound carbonic acid.

The use of coal-gas for lighting purposes is another common source of polluted atmosphere. By the combustion of 1 cubic foot of coal-gas, 2 cubic feet of carbonic acid are produced, and a considerable amount of sulphurous acid. A medium gas burner burns 3 cubic feet of gas per hour, and therefore produces as much carbonic acid as 10 individuals (6 cubic feet for one gas-burner as compared with ·6 cubic feet for one individual).

Effects of Breathing Impure Air.—The evil effects produced by expired air in a concentrated condition have been unhappily proved in a few well-known instances. In the Black Hole at Calcutta, 146 persons were confined in a space 18 feet every way, with two small windows on one side. Next morning 123 were found dead, and the remaining 23 were very ill. It must not be supposed, however, that no ill results follow a comparatively small degree of pollution, because these results are not immediately apparent. A general lowering of strength and vigour is produced, and a greater proneness to fall victim to respiratory and other diseases. The drowsiness and languor so frequently noticeable in school-children are, to the intelligent teacher, not an indication of wilful inattention, but of the necessity for a purer air. Yawning, again, is a cry of the nervous system for purer blood, *i.e.*, for blood containing more oxygen and less effete matters.

It is in the highest degree unfair to expect the brains of children to be in active exercise of their functions, while they are provided with blood which is vitiated by respiratory impurities, and are thus kept in a species of mental fog.

Children are especially susceptible to the dangers resulting from impure air. They are necessarily somewhat closely massed together, and the organic matters hanging about the room serve as a favourable soil for the propagation and development of infectious diseases, which in a pure air would soon lose their vitality. In this way diphtheria, scarlet fever, and like diseases are not uncommonly propagated at school. Tubercular consumption, again, has been clearly shown to be greatly favoured by over-crowding, and it is not impossible that its propagation from one child to another under such conditions does sometimes occur. In the case of rabbits and guinea-pigs, it is found that when they are kept in a small, close apartment for three months, tubercular disease is produced, and dogs under similar circumstances become consumptive.

Temperature of Air required.—The external temperature varies greatly with the season, and even at different parts of the same day. In Philadelphia the averages of ten years show that the mean temperature in the winter months is 33.2° Fahr., in spring 51.9°, in summer 76.1°, in autumn 55.7°. Now, the admission of air at 76° Fahr. makes a room uncomfortably warm, while the temperature of 32° could hardly be borne by the most robust of children. In one case, the entering air may with advantage be cooled; in the other, it must be warmed.

The temperature of each class-room should vary between 65° and 70° Fahr. In infant-schools the upper limit of 70° is preferable. Possibly a little higher than this would do no harm, but the heat-generating powers of the body are thus lowered, and the air is more likely to be vitiated.

Where hot-air or hot-water apparatus is the source of heat, a common experience is to begin the day in school with a temperature of 60°; but in a few hours, owing to deficient exit of impure air, and to the heat produced by the children themselves, the temperature has reached 70° or even 80° without being noticed, and now the children feel no warmer than when the thermometer stood at 60°. The excessive heat has produced a general languor of the circulation, and a dilated condition of the cutaneous blood-vessels, leading to a general lack of tone and vigour. For a similar reason the mental powers flag, and sleepiness is induced. Persons coming into the room from out-of-doors find the atmosphere intolerable, but the occupants, unfortunately, cannot judge for themselves. It is important that thermometers should be placed in conspicuous places in rooms (remote from the point of entry of hot air), and that their indication should be hourly ascertained. The remedy for a hot and close room is not to stop the further entry of warm fresh air, but to secure a freer escape of hot impure air.

Children, in the perspiring and low-toned condition produced by an over-heated room, are allowed to rush out into the cold corridors or offices of the school; and it is little wonder that quinsy, croup, bronchitis, and other troubles are frequently induced. The use of an alarm-thermometer, which would ring a bell as long as the temperature remained above 70°, would be very valuable.*

GENERAL PRINCIPLES OF VENTILATION. 27

Dryness of Air.—All air contains water in a gaseous condition, and the hotter the air the more water it will contain before the point of saturation is reached. For every increase of 27° in temperature, air doubles its capacity for holding water. The warm air supplied to school-rooms from heating appliances is often very dry. It then tends to abstract moisture from the skin and lungs, and produce a dry feverish condition, which is frequently noticeable in rooms heated by furnace or stove. A pail of water standing in the room, near the source of heat, helps to prevent this. It is doubtful whether, in many cases, the effects ascribed to dryness of air are not really due to escape of the products of combustion, such as carbonic oxide and sulphurous acid.

Amount of Air Required.—The limit of impurity of air beyond which it becomes perceptibly stuffy is ·06 per cent., or 6 parts in 10,000. In order to maintain the carbonic acid at this level, 3,000 cubic feet of pure air are required per hour by every adult, and more than half as much should be furnished for each scholar. This might be furnished by a large room with a slow circulation of air, or a small room with a rapid circulation of air. In a school-room the amount of space per child is necessarily limited; this must therefore be compensated for by a more frequent change of air.

The English Educational Department give 80 cubic feet as the minimum space per scholar, and 8 square feet as the minimum floor-space allowable. Under the London School Board, eight square feet per scholar are enforced in infant-schools. In senior schools the floor-space is calculated upon seat accommodation. This ensures on the whole slightly over 10 square feet of floor-space per child.

We may practically fix the permissible carbonic acid in the atmosphere of school-rooms as 1 part in 1,000, instead of the ideal limit of ·6 per 1,000; as it is doubtful if, with the 15 square tain 1,500 cubic feet of air per hour, it is evident that the air must be replaced at least every six minutes, *i.e.*, 10 times in an hour.

To recapitulate: the requirements of each class-room in a school building should not be less than 15 square feet of floor-area per pupil, and the window-space should equal one-fourth of the floor-space. Each pupil should be provided with 25 to 30 cubic feet of fresh air per minute, introduced and distributed without producing unpleasant draughts and having a temperature of from 60° to 65° Fahr.

The above represents the minimum of requirement for cold weather. In warm weather, as much fresh air must be introduced as open windows and doors will admit.

A fallacy frequently entertained is that deficiencies in floor-space may be compensated by a lofty ceiling. Such is not the case, however. A "lofty" room is not necessarily "airy." Any height above 12 feet has little or no influence on the purity of the lower atmosphere in which the children have to live; and cross-ventilation at a considerable height may leave the atmosphere of the lower level in which children breathe in a vitiated condition. It is not advisable to have school-rooms much higher than the windows, as warm and impure air tends to accumulate along the ceiling, subsequently falling to the floor-level as it cools.

CHAPTER VI.

Natural Ventilation.

Rules respecting Ventilation. — Natural and Artificial Ventilation.—Ventilation through Window, Wall, Chimney, and Ceiling.

Most treatises on ventilation and heating have been founded on European facts and figures, and are hence unreliable for the American climate. And even in speaking of the States alone, it is difficult to give general methods which shall be applicable to the great diversities of climate includ.d in its 25° of latitude, of which the only one feature in common is the inconstancy of the climate. New York, for instance, has been said to have the summer of Rome, and the winter of Copenhagen.

Ventilation is constantly being produced by two natural agencies, viz., the diffusion of gases, and the movements caused by differences of temperature.

Diffusion, by which the purer outside gases tend to mix with the impure internal air, is constantly going on, though the rate of diffusion is under ordinary circumstances slow and the amount of interchange thus effected is but small.

Differences of temperature cause much more active movements of air, warm air floating to the top of cold air, as oil floats to the top of water. The air in a room is warmed by the inmates and by the stove, gas, or other source of artificial heat. Cold air tends to rush in from every opening, and, being heavier than warm air, falls toward the floor, producing a draught. The great problem of ventilation is to secure a sufficient interchange of air without causing draughts. The entrance of air at any temperature below 50° into a room whose temperature is 65° or even 70° is almost certain to be accompanied by draught; hence it is necessary to warm the entering air during many of the winter months.

If a free entrance for pure air is not provided, the influence of the higher temperature in the school-room may produce an aspiration of air from undesirable places. Thus it not uncommonly happens that air is drawn from underground cellars, defective drains, water-closets, &c.

The following rules respecting ventilation are of importance:

(1.) The air should be drawn from a pure source.

(2.) No draught or current should be perceptible. Very often the remedy for a draught is not to close the opening, but to make others in order to increase the area through which air enters.

(3.) The entry of air should be constant, not at intervals.

(4.) An abundant exit for impure air should be provided separate from the points of entrance of fresh air. In order to maintain a given standard of purity, it is necessary to provide for the removal of as much impure air as is supplied of pure air.

Ventilation is of two kinds, natural and artificial. The first kind is produced by the ordinary interchange of air when windows or doors are allowed to remain open. Artificial ventilation is that produced by the extraneous help of heating apparatus or of mechanical appliances for propelling the air into a room or aspirating it from it.

Such mechanical measures are not practically useful for school-rooms, and we shall confine ourselves to the consideration of ventilation by natural means and by heating apparatus.

Natural Ventilation is possible as an exclusive plan only during the summer months. In colder weather the admission of external air produces violent draughts. Any reliance on it as the source of pure air is practically found to end in the careful closure of all windows, doors, and ventilating apertures, and a resulting foulness of atmosphere which is only too common in school-rooms.

When the external temperature reaches 60°, or better still 65°, the air may be freely admitted. Open *windows* are by far the best means of ventilation, and during the school recess all the windows should be thrown open, opposite windows if possible or doors and windows, in order that the rooms may be thoroughly flushed with air. Ordinary ventilation commonly leaves a considerable proportion of organic volatile matter from respiration hanging about the room, while the rapid currents of air during the flushing of a room carry this away.

The occurrence of any down-draught from an open window may be prevented by having its upper segment made to work on a hinge, lateral triangular pieces of glass being inserted on each side of the window (Fig. 4) ; or a narrow piece of wood may be

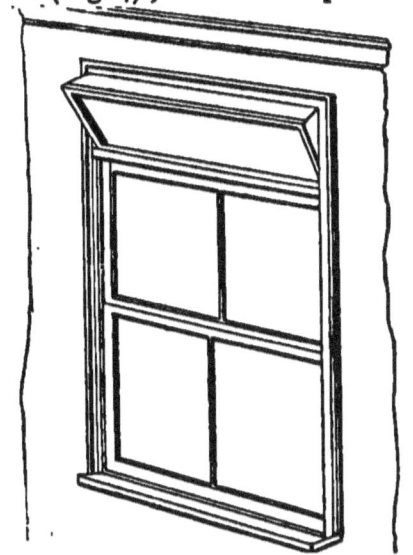

4.—Diagram of ventilation by hinged windows.

inserted under the lower sash of the window, an upward current of air being thus allowed between the two sashes. (Fig. 5.)

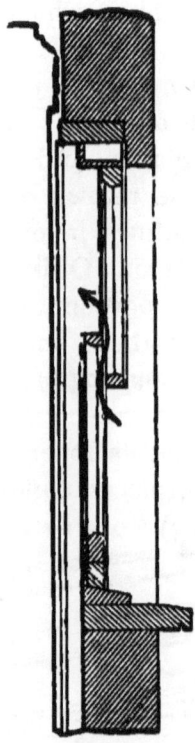

FIG. 5.—Ventilation between window-sashes, a block being fitted under the lower sash.

Sometimes the top sash is opened and wire gauze is fastened across, but by this plan the amount of air which enters is much less than through a continuous opening of the same area.

The *wall* may be utilised for ventilating purposes by the insertion of a grating near the floor which is connected on its inner aspect to a vertical tube, an upward direction being thus given to the entering air. (Fig. 6) Or the grating may be placed higher up, a movable valve on the inner side of the wall directing the current upwards. (Fig. 7.)

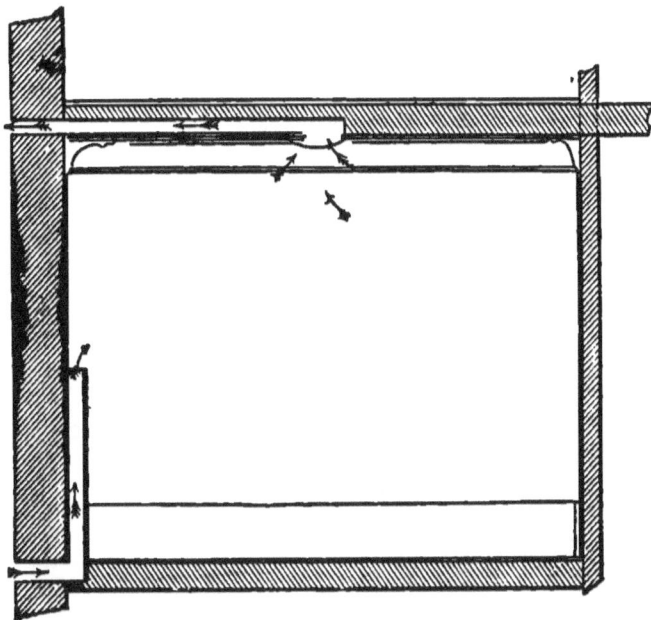

FIG. 6.—Diagram showing ventilation by Tobin's tube, and an exit-shaft leading from centre-flower of ceiling.

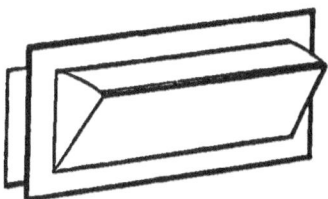

FIG. 7.—Sheringham's ventilator.

The ventilation is much more likely to be successful if there are openings on opposite sides of the room, or if there is a chimney or other draught-compeller, in the school-room.

Indeed a *chimney* should always be allowed for each room, even when it is not contemplated to have open fires. Owing to the aspirating effect of winds acting at the top of the chimney, there is generally an up-current, and always so if there is free ingress of air by doors or windows. The action of the chimney in withdrawing impure air from a room, may be greatly increased by narrowing its two ends, so as to produce a more rapid current at the entrance and exit of air.

Flap's or Arnott's valves (Fig. 8) placed above the fireplace and opening into the flue, are of some service in withdrawing hot impure air collected near the ceiling, though the extent of their value must not be over-estimated, as the amount of air passing through them is, on account of their size, necessarily limited.

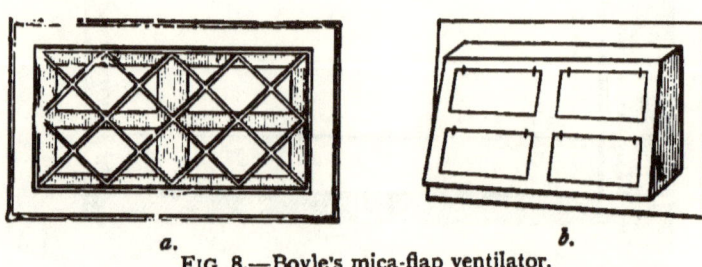

FIG 8.—Boyle's mica-flap ventilator.
a, View from room.   *b*, View from chimney.

The *ceiling* may be utilised for carrying off foul air, and as the foul air from respiration is warm, it rises to the top of the room, and may with advantage be at once removed.

A grating in the external wall may be made to correspond to the space between the ceiling and the floor of the room next above, and apertures in the ceiling made to communicate with this. (Fig. 6.) Or an air-tight zinc chamber between the ceiling and the room above may be carried, by means of a zinc pipe, into the chimney, the junction with the latter being guarded by a valve working only in one direction.

The use of ventilating gas-burners should always be enforced, the products of the combustion of gas being thus at once removed, and at the same time much impure air from the room. (Fig 3, page 20.) It is important, however, that children should not work in a room where gas is required during the day, and that their evening studies should be very short.

In order that natural ventilation may be more effectual, all corridors should be large and airy, and have windows opening direct to the outer air. No school-plan which does not fulfil these conditions can be regarded as satisfactory.

In the methods of ventilation hitherto described, the air is admitted at the same temperature as the external air. Such methods have, however, but a limited application in the States. During a large portion of the year, in order to prevent dangerous draughts, the incoming air requires warming. The means by which the incoming air can be warmed will be discussed in the next chapter.

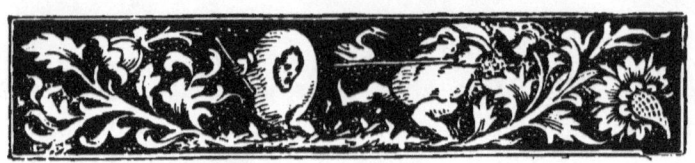

CHAPTER VII.

VENTILATION AND WARMING.

Difficulties of Successful Ventilation by Warm Air.—Open Fireplace.—Heating by Gas.—Closed Stoves.—Central System of Heating.—Hot-Air Furnaces.—Steam Apparatus.—Hot-Water Apparatus.—Entrance Flues and Extraction Shafts.—The Bridgeport System.

A DOUBLE heading has been purposely made to this chapter. In fact, ventilation and warming, to be in accordance with the laws of health, always require to be conjointly considered. A successful system of warming a school must necessarily, for purposes of health, provide pure air; and a successful system of ventilation must, at least in the winter months, also furnish warmth.

These considerations bring us face to face with the serious question of *expense*. The warming of a large volume of air means the expenditure of coal or gas, and ventilation means the discharge of this *warmed and therefore expensive* air as soon as it becomes impure. If, in order to diminish expense, no provision is made for the escape of the warm air as it becomes polluted, the school-room speedily becomes foul and unhealthy, —a very hot-bed of disease.

When the necessary expensiveness of ventilation is fairly grasped by school-managers, surely there will be an end of the economising over ventilation which is now so general. Such economising is most certainly at the expense of the children's health, and tends yearly to greatly increase our bill of mortality.

No system of warming and ventilation has been devised which will work automatically without the supervision of a competent officer. Brains are required as well as coal and an apparatus for this purpose; a watchful and intelligent supervision to see that the temperature and the ingress and egress of air are properly adjusted.

The school-keeper, who is generally responsible for the maintenance of hot-air apparatus, not uncommonly regards ventilation as inimical to his interests, and will, in case the heat is lowered, stop the valves leading to the exit-flues, thus penning up the hot impure air, rather than apply the extra fuel required. It is to his interest to appear economical of coal; he is, therefore, under the constant temptation to check the outflow of warm air from the rooms, and to minimise the period of flushing them with external air after school hours.

The system of warm-air ventilation to be used will vary with the size of the school and with local conditions. For small schools some of the following plans may be adopted, though in large schools a central system is the best.

The Open Fire-place not only furnishes a cheerful warmth, but is likewise a valuable purifier of the atmosphere of a room, as from 14,000 to 20,000 cubic feet of air pass up an ordinary chimney each hour. Thus, reckoning 1,500 cubic feet for each scholar, the respiratory impurities of from 9 to 13 scholars can be got rid of in this way. The open fire-place, however, does not form a convenient source of heat except for small rooms, for the following reasons :—(1) The heat is unequally distributed, being, for instance, 9 times as great at a distance of one foot from the fire as it is at a distance of 3 feet. (2) Currents of cold air are produced along the floor in order to supply the place of the air which is rushing up the chimney. These are very trying unless a free supply of warm air from some other source than the fire is allowed. (3) There is the trouble of frequently replenishing the fire, interfering with studies.

The great loss of heat necessarily involved in an open fire-place has led to the use of chambers behind the fire-place, by which external air is warmed as it enters the room. A stove constructed on this principle is shown in Fig. 9. At the back of the stove is an air-chamber communicating with the external air.

Air admitted through the opening (*a*, Fig. 9) is warmed by coming in contact with the fire-clay (*d*), which separates the air-channel from the smoke flue (*c*). The warmed air leaves the air-channel by the grating (*b*) over the fire-place, and then travels along the upper part of the room, falling to the floor as it cools and finally escaping up the chimney.

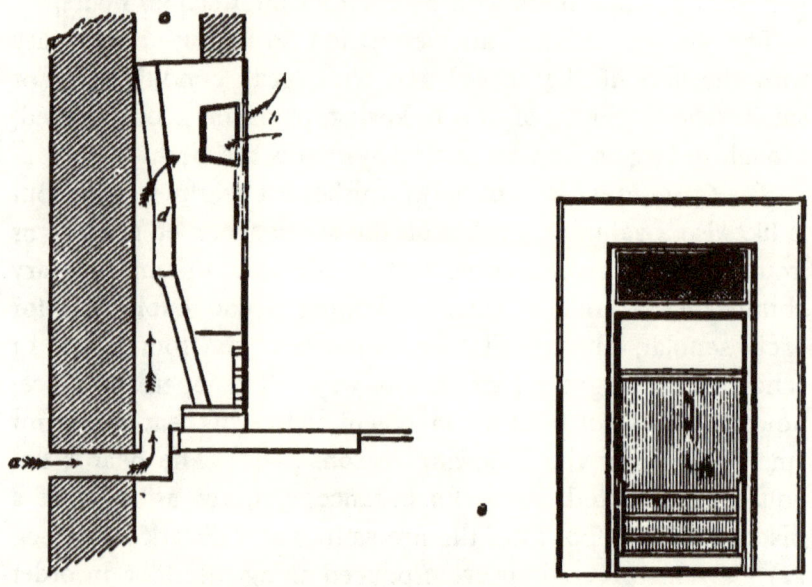

FIG. 9.—Slow-combustion ventilating stove.
1.—Section of stove, showing—*a*, entrance of cold air; *b*, entrance of warmed air into room; *c*, smoke-flue; *d*, fireclay back of stove.
2.—Front elevation of same stove.

VENTILATION AND WARMING. 39

Gas is sometimes employed instead of coal for fires.

No gas-stove should be allowed in which provision is not made for carrying off all the products of combustion. A chimney or pipe for carrying away the gases produced is even more necessary than in the case of a coal-fire, for in the latter case the smoke produced would necessitate a recourse to open windows or other means of ventilation, while in the former the deleterious products are invisible. Gas is suitable as a means of heating only small rooms, owing to its greater expense. Several stoves are convenient and thoroughly sanitary; they are placed in an open fire-place with a flue-pipe attached. For school-rooms where gas is, for special reasons, employed as the heating agent, the Calorigen stove is a valuable means of supplying warm and pure air. Its arrangement is shown in Fig. 10. A spiral tube communicates below with the

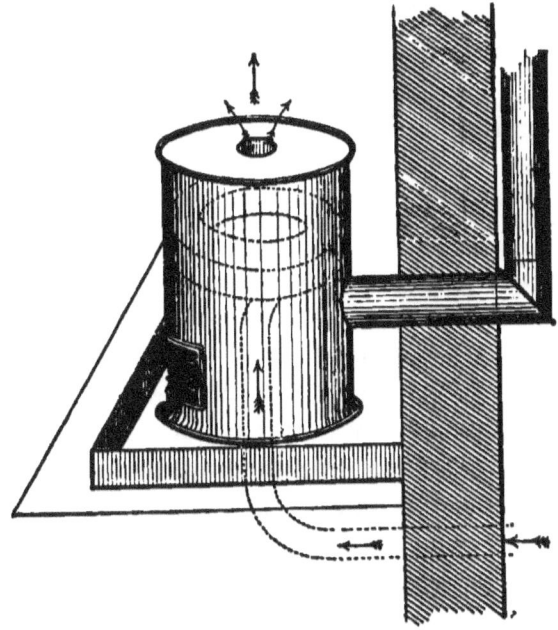

FIG. 10.—The Calorigen stove.

external air, and opens at its upper end into the room. A small gas-flame is kept burning below the spiral tube, the products of combustion from which are carried directly out-of-doors. The heat thus produced warms the air which is passing along the spiral tube and causes a constant rapid entry of warm air into the room.

Closed Stoves are useful chiefly in small school-rooms, either gas or coal being burnt. They possess the advantage over an open fire-place, that there is a smaller consumption of fuel, and that the combustion can be more effectually regulated. Commonly, however, they make the air of a room dry, and produce a peculiar close smell, probably owing to the charring of minute organic particles. It is found also that carbonic oxide may pass through cracks or even through the substance of iron stoves, when they are red-hot. When stoves are employed, firebrick should be everywhere in contact with the fire, and the stove should never be allowed to become red-hot. There should be as few joints as possible, and these should be horizontal and not vertical. The supply of air to the stove should never be cut off, nor should the escape of the products of combustion be prevented by dampers, or by admitting air between the stove and the chimney.

We are strongly of opinion that stoves should be allowed only in combination with some provision for warming the incoming air. This may be secured by having a sheet iron or zinc cylinder, considerably wider than the stove-pipe, placed round it and fastened to the floor below. A good-sized pipe is then carried through the floor and out to the external wall of the school. In this way a large supply of warmed air is drawn into the room (Fig. 11). Similarly the stove-pipe may be utilised by enclosing it in another pipe, which starts some distance from the stove, and is carried into the chimney. This causes the abstraction of considerable impure air. If required, impure air may be withdrawn from the next room below by a modification of this method.

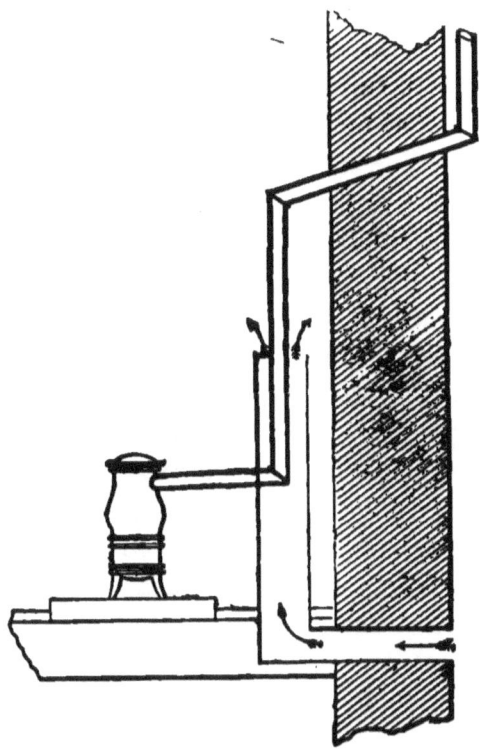

FIG. 11.—Closed stove arranged to warm incoming fresh-air.

Central System of Heating.—Hot air, steam, and hot water are the usual sources of heat employed, and each plan will require consideration.

The great majority of *Hot-air Furnaces* are unsatisfactory for several reasons.—(1.) The furnace is generally too small; consequently, in severely cold weather, the radiating surfaces are unduly heated and the joints may be loosened. Carbonic oxide and sulphurous acid may then escape, the latter being fortunately irritant, but the former odourless and recognised only by the giddiness, languor, and peculiar discomfort produced. Carbonic oxide will pass through red-hot cast-iron, but the danger from the sand-holes produced in defective casting, or from badly-fitting joints, is probably much greater. Wrought-iron furnaces do not allow the escape of carbonic oxide through their substance, but the joints may crack; and wrought-iron oxidises more rapidly than cast-iron.

(2.) No provision is made for mixing cool with the heated air, which is often distributed at 140°. To cool the room the register is shut off, the poor scholars being then obliged to rebreathe the same atmosphere repeatedly.

(3.) The source of the air supply to the furnace is often most unsatisfactory. The furnace-room may contain decomposing vegetables or an empty bell-trap leading to a defective drain or a water-closet, none of which increase the purity of the school atmosphere. If the furnace-room is underground, it is not infrequently kept closed, and then the air which is warmed may be the air already breathed by the scholars, and subsequently drawn down into the cellar. A large furnace is best, as it never needs to be made red-hot. It should have the fewest joints and the largest amount of radiating-surface, in proportion to the size of the fire-box, that can be secured.

Steam Apparatus is perhaps more frequently used than any other in the United States; and it offers such great advantages, that it is to be regretted that it is not more frequently used in other countries. It is much more easily made to work and is cheaper than hot-water apparatus, and there is less difficulty in planning it. Also the radiating surfaces, being at a higher temperature than with hot water, may be made smaller and more compact.

Its chief disadvantages are that (1) constant attention is required to keep up the supply of heat, as the radiating surfaces cool much more rapidly than hot-water apparatus. (2) The radiators being at a very high temperature it is difficult to regulate the supply of heat in accordance with the outdoor temperature.

This may be remedied by arranging each set of radiators in several different sections, in each of which the flow of steam can be regulated independently of the others. Or the air ducts and flues may be so arranged that by movement of a valve the air can be made to pass wholly in contact with the radiating surfaces or separate from them in any proportion. Such a plan requiries the superintendence of a skilled attendant.

Hot-water Apparatus possesses some advantages over steam-apparatus, in the facts that the air passing over hot-water pipes is as a rule not raised above 100° F., with a temperature of the pipes of from 160-180°, and that hot water continues to circulate some time after the fire is extinguished.

We shall mention only to condemn the system of "*Direct Radiation*," in which steam-pipes are placed in a room without any provision for the entry of warmed air. This has been well described as "one of the most killing systems in existence." The use of hot-water pipes (apart from arrangements for ventilation), whether on the low-pressure or high-pressure system, is similarly to be condemned. In every case provision should be made for passing the cold external air over the pipes as it enters the room.

In discussing the preceding systems of warming, we have assumed that warmed air is admitted in amount proportionate to the number of scholars. Each scholar requiries 1,500 cubic feet of air per hour; therefore, assuming the space per head as 150 cubic feet, it follows that the air of the room must be replenished every 6 minutes. At the same time an equal (or slightly larger) amount of air must be removed to make way for the pure air.

Suppose we have to arrange for a school with from 8 to 12

class-rooms, each with 40 to 60 pupils, and that these are in connection with a large central hall in a two-story brick building. Ordinarily, architects concern themselves entirely with the provision of extraction-shafts for foul air, trusting for pure air to what can enter through slits in the window-sills, &c., while the heating-apparatus is apart from any ventilation.

The provision of these extraction-shafts is of great importance, and we may consider them first. As a rule there should be an aspirating shaft or chimney on each side of the central hall. A room containing 50 scholars, should discharge 2 ; cubic feet of air per second ; a flue carrying air with a velocity of 6 feet per second should therefore be 2 feet square, exclusive of the space allowed for smoke-flue or other heating apparatus. (Dr. Billings.) Such extraction, however, without the provision of warm pure air to take its place, is never satisfactory. The *vis a tergo* as well as the *vis a fronte* is required in order to maintain a pure atmosphere. The system adopted at the High School, Bridgeport, Connecticut, is one of the most successful and complete hitherto adopted, as it fulfils all the requirements of school ventilation and warming. (For details see 3rd Annual Report of Connecticut State Board of Health.)

In this system the coil-boxes heated by steam are placed on the inner wall, extensive piping being thus saved and the danger of freezing obviated. Fresh air is passed through the coil-chambers and conveyed to the rooms by metallic flues entering the inner wall about 8 feet from the floor. Thence it diffuses itself along the walls and ceiling, passing down the opposite wall and returning at a lower level to the flue for exit of impure air, which is placed under a platform measuring 6 by 12 feet on movable castors and on the same side of the room as the introduction-flue.

Careful experiments have shown that no other relative position of entrance and exit flues ensures so thorough and equable a warming of the room, and replenishing of its atmosphere. The entire lower edge of the platform is 4 inches from the floor, to allow full circulation of air under it.

In order that a strong up-current may be constantly ensured in the foul-air shafts, other coils are placed in them, and the entrance and boiler flues are also made to pass through the foul-air shafts, of course without any communication. The foul-air or extraction shafts should never be placed in the outer wall if possible, owing to the defective up-current from loss of heat. If such an arrangement cannot be avoided, the loss of heat may be diminished by a double wall and air space.

The difficulty of regulating the temperature of the rooms without closing the registers has been overcome in the Bridgeport School-house, by enclosing the heating surface for each room in a separate jacket of metal and then subdividing it into five sections, so arranged that any number may be used or cut off at pleasure, the supply of pure air remaining always the same.

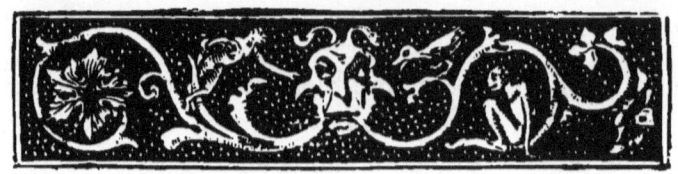

CHAPTER VIII.

DRAINAGE ARRANGEMENTS.

Lavatories. — *Urinals.* — *Water-closets.* — *Soil-pipe.* — *Drains.* — *Earth-closets.*

THE school premises should always be so placed that there is a fall from them capable of being utilised for drainage. A site without means of drainage is not worth having at any price.

Lavatories should be kept strictly clean, and the waste-pipes not allowed to run directly into the drain, but trapped, with a fresh-air inlet on the house side of the trap. In one case, the writer distinctly traced an outbreak of typhoid fever in a school to the direct connection of the lavatory-waste with a Mansergh's trap, the arrangement of which had been inverted by an ignorant workman. In cold climates, disconnection, on the English system, is impracticable. It is well to remember that sometimes the overflow-pipes from wash-basins are connected with the drain, even when the waste-pipes are properly disconnected. An offensive smell may arise from decomposing soap in lavatory waste-pipes; hence, when several basins are connected with a common waste-pipe, the angles of junction should be very obtuse. In addition, the waste-pipe from each basin should have a syphon-bend close under the basin, to prevent offensive smells from decomposing soap in the waste pipe, and a ventilating pipe from this to prevent the water in the bend being exhausted by syphon-action. (Fig. 12.) The preceding plan is the best where there is not frequent danger of the water freezing in the gully-trap. (*b*, Fig. 12.) In the States, however, this is so common an event in winter that the

DRAINAGE ARRANGEMENTS. 47

gully-trap has to be abandoned; and the lavatory waste-pipe must be directly connected with other waste-pipes which discharge into the drain. In this case the syphon-bend shown at *c*, and the ventilation shaft shown at *d*, must be insisted on. (Fig. 12.)

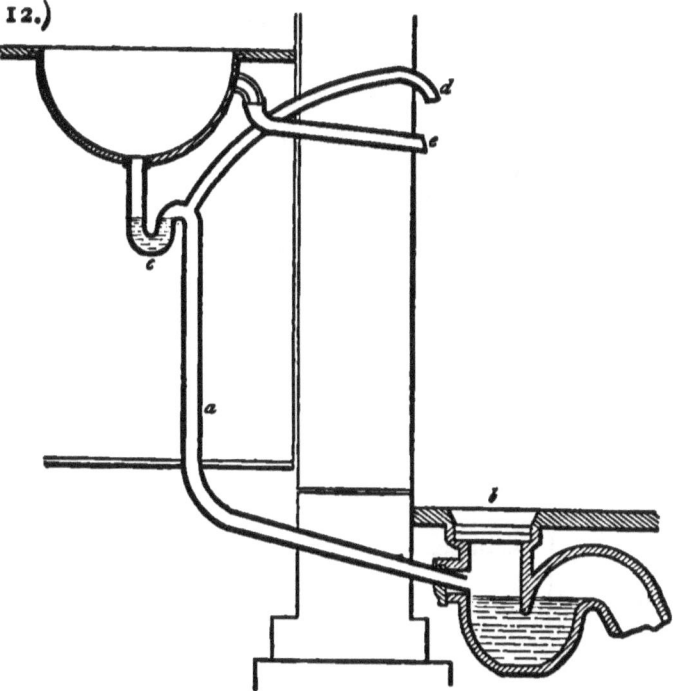

FIG 12.—Lavatory wash-basin.

a, Waste-pipe, emptying over water-seal of gully-trap (*b*); *c*, syphon-trap in waste-pipe to prevent foul-air from waste-pipe getting into room; *d*, ventilating pipe from syphon to prevent unsyphoning; *e*, discharge of overflow pipe.

Urinals are best furnished with china or glazed earthenware pans, as these hardly allow any sediment. Slate, stone, or cement slabs should not be used, as the rougher surface allows deposit, and they can be written on. Water should not be allowed to trickle down for cleansing purposes, as children play with it, and even try to drink. Frequent washing by an attendant is best, or the provision of an automatic flush-tank, which discharges its contents at intervals. Five places for each hundred children are required. The waste-pipe from the urinal should open into a ventilated trap, and not be directly connected with the drain.

Closets should never be placed in the basement under the school. They may be partially connected with the school by a covered subway, but should always be in a separate building. The walls of the closet should be of a material that cannot be written on, tiles being best for this purpose, and all closets should be frequently inspected. The proper allowance is one seat for every 15 girls or 25 boys (or less), the seats being proportionate to the children's stature, and the closets divided by partitions. There should be separate provision for teachers and the two sexes.

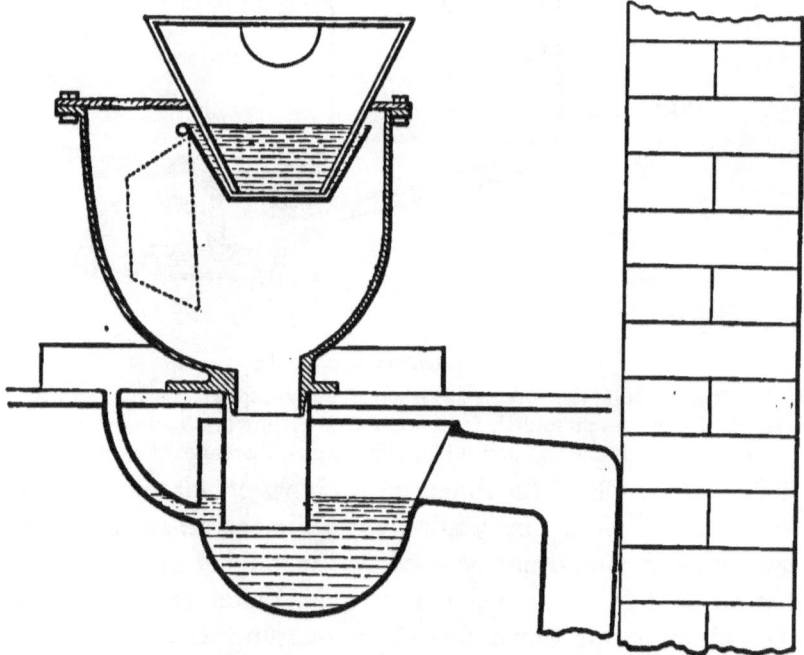

FIG. 13.—Pan closet, with D trap beneath.
An illustration of the form of closet most commonly used, but most dangerous to health.

DRAINAGE ARRANGEMENTS. 49

The common privy is most objectionable from a sanitary standpoint. Either water or earth closets should be employed. Of water-closets, pan-closets are always bad, and simple

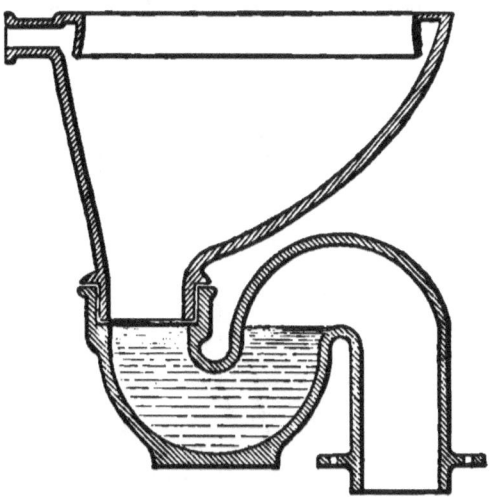

FIG. 14.—An improved hopper closet.

valveless closets are most suitable. The water supply should be abundant, and from a cistern distinct from that supplying drinking-water. The amount of fall from the cistern to the closet should be at least 3 or 4 feet, and the internal diameter of the flushing-pipe at least $1\frac{1}{4}$ inch. For teachers' closets, the valve closet shown in Fig. 15 is a very good form, especially where such a closet is in the main building near class-rooms. As lifting a handle is required for flushing purposes, it should never be allowed for children, for whom the valveless closet shown in Fig. 14 is most suitable, combined with an automatic flushing arrangement, worked by rising from the seat.

Instead of isolated water-closets, the *tumbler-closet* or *trough-closet* may be employed, each having a number of seats and a water-tight trough below, the contents of which are emptied only at intervals by a flush of water, and the removal of a plug. It carefully superintended, such an arrangement works fairly well; but if neglected, a considerable nuisance is produced.

The soil-pipe should be carried above the roof of the

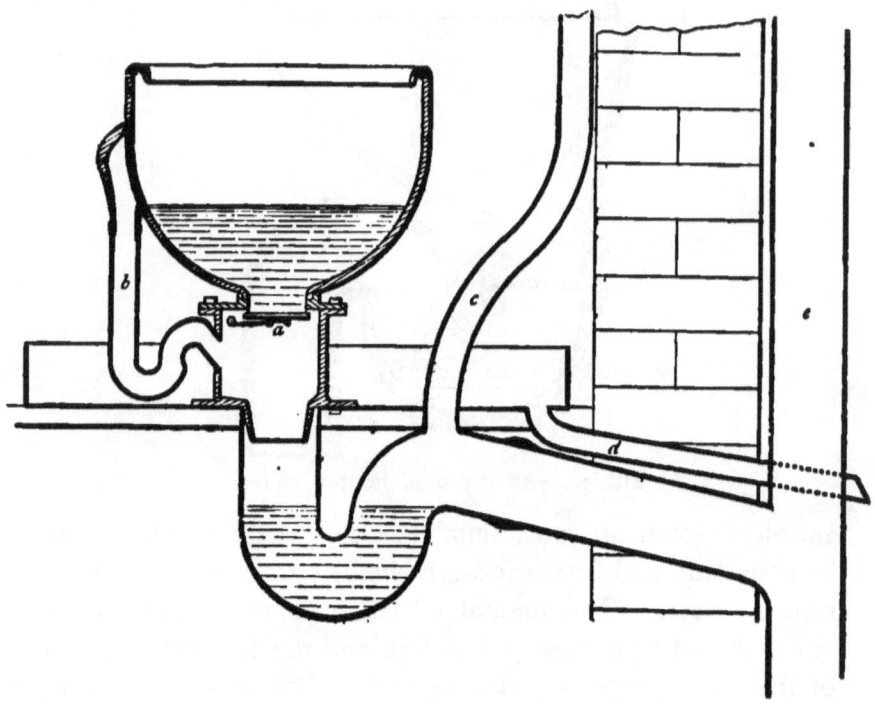

FIG. 15. — A sanitary valve-closet.

a, valve which is opened by a handle; *b*, overflow pipe from pan of closet; *c*, small ventilating-pipe connected with syphon-trap to prevent its being emptied of water by syphon-action (it is carried through the wall a little higher up); *d*, waste-pipe from tray to catch accidental spillings, made to discharge beyond the outer wall, and not connected with soil-pipe; *e*, ventilating-shaft continued upward from soil-pipe.

school-building, with a wire grating over the top, and a ventilated trap placed at the other end of the school drain-

DRAINAGE ARRANGEMENTS.

age system, thus insuring complete ventilation of the school-drain.

The Drain-pipe should be as small as is consistent with its carrying away all waste matters. The larger it is, the more liable it is to become blocked. Iron pipes are preferable to brick or earthenware, especially within the house. They should be coated inside and out with some material which completely withstands all chemical action and changes of temperature.

The drain-pipe should be separated from the main sewer by a syphon-trap which is ventilated, thus allowing fresh air to sweep from one end of the school drainage system to the other.

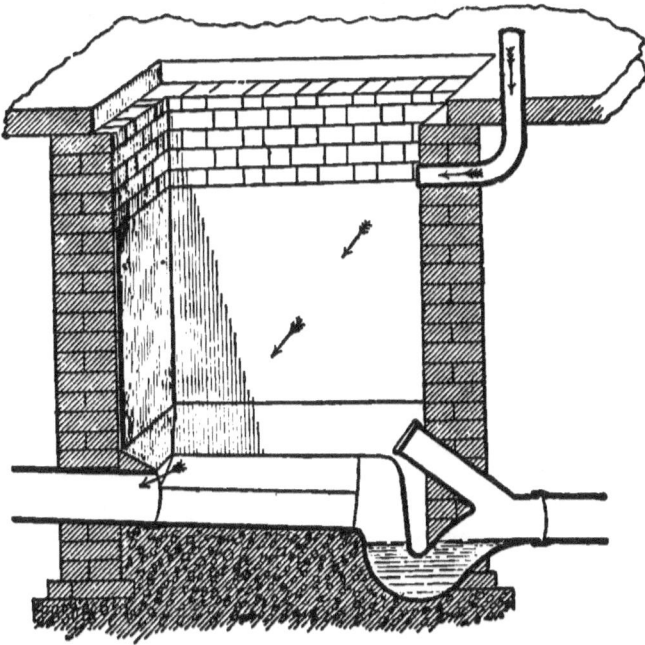

FIG. 16.—Vertical section of disconnecting-chamber with intercepting trap, showing ventilation of school-drain and method of reaching pipes for cleansing purposes.

Under no circumstances should a *cesspool*, "the king of nuisances," be allowed to receive the school-drainage. It

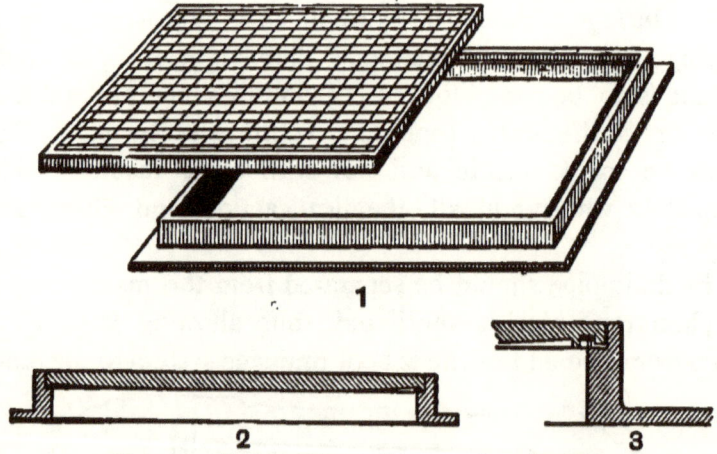

Fig. 17.—Iron cover to disconnecting-chamber.

1, The iron cover removed. 2, Section of cover and frame. 3, India-rubber seating at angle, forming an air-tight junction.

forms a manufactory for poisonous sewer-gases, even more effectually than a badly-constructed sewer. The soil around the cesspool tends to become "excrement-sodden," and the water of any well in the neighbourhood is in constant danger of contamination.

Children are apt to play or hide about retired parts of the school-ground, and thus may be endangered by the effluvia from the cesspool.

When there is no central system of drainage, *Earth-closets* should always be used, and, even when this is available, earth-closets present a great advantage in the absence of fear of the water-supply becoming frozen. It is found that $1\frac{1}{2}$lb. of dry, loamy earth will completely deodorise the closet each time it is used. The earth must be dry. It has been well said by Moule, the originator of the system, that "an earth closet will no more work without *dry* earth, than a water-closet will work without water." Pure sand and gravel or chalk are nearly useless, but sawdust answers fairly well.

When earth-closets are adopted, the waste water from lavatories and urinals requires separate treatment. In country places the best plan is to collect the waste water in an automatic flush-tank, which, when it becomes full, discharges all its contents into loosely-laid drains under the surface of a garden or field. In this way the water is effectually discharged at intervals, while at the same time a sodden condition of the soil is not produced.

PART II.

SCHOLARS.

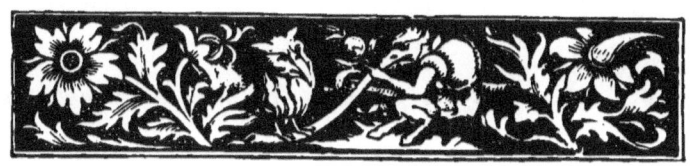

CHAPTER IX.

Mental Exercise.

Full Scope of Education.—Quantity and Quality of Brain.—The Brain a Compound Organ.—Functional Habits of Brain.—Blood Supply.—Sensory and Muscular Education of Brain.

It cannot be too clearly understood that the function of education is to prepare a child for his after-life, and the true test of the value of an educational course lies in whether it fulfils this end. In order that the preparation may be complete, the physical, mental, and moral parts of a child's nature must be embraced within its scope. A lack of education in any one of these, leads to the production of an ill-balanced and defective manhood. These parts of our nature are inextricably associated, and defects in one react injuriously on the others. It is unfortunate that so very narrow a view of the scope of education is usually taken. That is the best schooling which most completely prepares a child for his future career, by training his powers of observation, memory, and reflection, while at the same time imparting knowledge which shall be of practical service in life.

Physical education we shall discuss in Chap. XII.; here we are chiefly concerned with mental education in its bearings on health.

Whatever view of the relation of mind and brain be taken

it will be agreed that the brain is the instrument necessary to all mental operations.

The exercise of the brain involved in education leads to an increase in its size and an improvement in its quality beyond what occurs in the uneducated. The average weight of the brain in the adult European is between 49 and 50 ounces. In civilised races it is heavier than in the less civilised, and even in the highly-civilised races an increase in the size of the brain has occurred in historic times.

At birth the weight of the brain averages from 11 to 14 ounces, and a progressive increase, most rapid in the earlier years, occurs, the greatest average weight of the male brain being reached at the age of 35, and of the female brain at about 30.

Just as increased muscular exercise leads to increased size and strength of the muscles, so may increased brain-exercise, during the period of its natural growth, accelerate and increase the individual growth of brain, and lead to the transmission of a tendency to larger brains.

Size of brain is not the only consideration, for the brain of a child seven years old is equal to nine-tenths of its weight in the adult, and at three years it is equal to three-fourths of the full weight. Nevertheless, other things being equal, the man with the largest brain has the greatest chance of success.

The *quality* of the structure of a brain, and the *degree of elaboration* of its grey matter, have also to be considered; and they vary much, even in brains of equal size. Education doubtless elaborates the structure of a brain, and multiplies connections between its cells, as well as probably increasing the number of cells.

The brain must hardly be considered as a single organ, but *a collection of organs*, which, although most intimately united, are also capable in some degree of independent action.

Different convo'u ions of the brain have been proved by Hitzig and Ferrier to have special functions, and it is probable that excessive development of any one faculty is accompanied by a disproportionate development of a corresponding convolution. The importance of early and systematic exercise directed to the uniform development of all parts of the brain, cannot be exaggerated. A genius in one direction should not be allowed too early to follow its own bent, or an ill-balanced mind is the inevitable consequence. There is some degree of truth in the statement that there is but a step between the ill-balanced brain of a genius and that of a lunatic.

Studies requiring observation, memory, or reasoning-power, bring into action different parts of the brain, and should all in turn receive careful and balanced attention. If the emotions are allowed to have a preponderant influence, life becomes wavering and uncontrolled by the will; while in some logically-minded individuals the emotions seem to have no place.

The u ility of a brain depends largely on its *functional habits*. Corresponding to each thought, there is probably a nerve-current in a particular part of the brain. Currents of nerve-force travel preferably in the pathways of least resistance, and these are where currents have repeatedly passed. Careful and persevering attention to special points will thus strengthen individual character, and may even lead to the formation of new mental habits. In this way it may be possible to counteract evil hereditary tendencies, and, by the aid of a wise teacher, to form a strong and evenly-balanced mind.

The brain is dependent for the continuance of its functions on an abundant and pure *supply of blood*. Any mental excitement causes a determination of blood to the brain. The more the brain is exercised within reasonable limits, the more blood it receives, and consequently the more it grows. If one part of the brain is disproportionately exercised, it grows disproportionately, while if the exercise is excessive other evils may be produced. (See Chap. X.)

Deficient food, indigestion, or an impure atmosphere, causes listlessness, apathy, headache, and other nervous symptoms, owing to impoverishment of the brain by deficient blood, or poisoning of it by impure blood.

The brain is not only the organ of thought and volition and the emotions, but is also the centre for the reception of impressions from other parts of the body and the external world, and the interpretation of these.

The influence of sensory and muscular impressions on the brain is so important as to call for some further remarks.

Sensations are perceived as such in the brain, the sensory organ (eye, ear, etc.) simply serving as a receptive medium which conveys the external stimulus to the brain.

The different sensations are received in separate parts of the brain. The resultant of these sensations stored up in the brain constitutes memory. It is evident that the cultivation of one sensory organ (or rather of the corresponding part of the brain) may be encouraged to the neglect of other senses, and thus an ill-balanced condition produced. For instance, a boy may have an excellent sense of touch, or an accurate perception of weight and resistance, and yet have no taste for music. Each sense requires special cultivation, and becomes skilled in proportion to the education received. It has been well said by Dr. Clarke : " If a single organ is wanting, or a single function not performed, just so much less brain development results." It is also unhappily true that the imperfect performance of any one mental function reacts injuriously on others. Hence the truth of the poetical statement—

" Break but one
Of a thousand keys, and the paining jar
Through all will run."—(Whittier.)

When the education of the senses is neglected, all subsequent education has a haziness about it which is almost irremediable. The Kindergarten system, cultivating the senses and powers of observation and construction from the earliest period, is of great value in this connection.

The brain controls and commands all voluntary *muscular movements*. In doing this, the motor part of the brain is necessarily exercised. In this way, gymnastics exercise the brain and increase its size. If an arm is amputated or paralysed in infancy, there is so much less brain in the adult. The influence of muscular exercise on brain-development will be further discussed in Chap. XII.

Brain-exercise is not carried on solely in our schools. It commences at the earliest period of life, and never ceases throughout conscious existence.

In the early years of life, the sensory, motor, and observing portions of the brain are chiefly exercised; while the exercise of the reasoning-powers and memory is that with which teachers are chiefly concerned. We must again repeat, however, that any education which does not bring into healthful and balanced action every part of a child's nature cannot be regarded as satisfactory or complete.

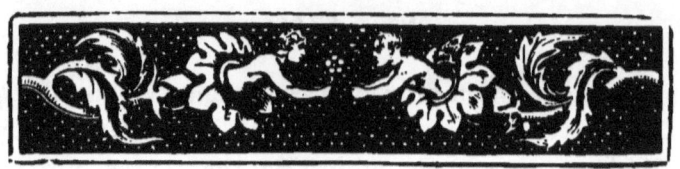

CHAPTER X.

Excessive Mental Exercise.

Symptoms and Effects of Brain-forcing.—The " Cram" System.— Causes of Over-strain —Home Lessons.—Badly arranged Work.— Importance of Technical Instruction.—Good and Bad Examinations.—Consumption from Over-work.—Punishments.

THE general raising of the standard of education and the fact that it is becoming universal, render the danger of excessive mental exercise increasingly great.

An adult brain in the intervals of work has to repair its structural losses and lay up a store of potential energy for future use ; the brain during the period of school-life has *also* to build up fresh material for its growth.

If we obtain mental maturity at an early age, it is at the expense of stability and real power. The higher the organism the longer it takes to arrive at maturity, is a biological law the truth of which is shown by the fact that precocity is generally followed by inferior mental organisation. Striking exceptions to this rule will doubtless occur to the reader, but the truth of it in ordinary cases is fairly established.

The evils of a vicious system of education were long ago depicted by Charles Dickens. " Dr. Blimber's establishment was a great hot-house in which there was a forcing-apparatus constantly at work. Mental green-peas were produced at

Christmas, and intellectual asparagus all the year round. Nature was of no consequence at all; no matter what a young gentleman was intended to bear, Dr. Blimber made him bear to order somehow or other. This was very pleasant and ingenious, but the system of forcing was attended with its usual disadvantages; there was not a right taste about the premature productions, and they didn't keep well. . . . And people did say that the Doctor had rather overdone it with young Toots, who, when he had whiskers, left off having brains."

Ordinary school-work, interrupted by vacations, seldom produces excessive strain on the mental powers of children. It is only in exceptional cases, where the children are insufficiently fed, or are of a peculiarly excitable temperament, or where the hours of study are unduly prolonged, that this result is likely to ensue. Such over-strain may also occur when one particular class of work is persisted in to excess, to the exclusion of varied work and of recreative exercise.

In such cases, *headache* is one of the first symptoms to attract attention. The parent is a much better judge as to whether the school-work is overtaxing the child, than the teacher, as the latter has to deal with a large class and can scarcely watch with sufficient care each child. If a child frequently complains of headache, it may be due to overwork, though the far more frequent causes—such as indigestion, bad atmosphere, defects of vision—should first be eliminated.

Many children seem indolent and stupid in school. The proper remedy for this, in not a few cases, is not some form of punishment, but attention to the general state of health, or sometimes a relaxation of studies. In some cases, apparent stupidity is really due to some defect of vision, a form of "artificial stupidity" which is discussed in Chap. XVII.

The brain may, in rare cases, become congested from overwork, and in certain cases, where a strong tubercular tendency exists, this would tend to produce meningitis (brain-fever). It would be unfair, however, to ascribe tubercular meningitis directly to school-work, as it is common both before and after the school-period of life. The school-work (like any other form of excitement) might tend to hasten such an attack.

Dr. Sturges, in the *Lancet* (Jan. 3, 1885), gives 200 cases of chorea (St. Vitus's dance), of which 79 were of known causation, and 14 of these, or 1 in 6, were apparently due to schooling. Doubtless the 14 should be taken from a larger number than 79, and the fact that chorea in children who do not attend school, occurs chiefly in the school-period of life, must be remembered.

Dr. McLane Hamilton's recent investigations show that over 20 per cent. of the young children in the public schools of New York have choreic affections of greater or less gravity.

Chorea is a disease rather of the poor than of the rich, so under-feeding may be a factor in its production. Very often a sudden shock, as from a severe whipping or a fright, is the cause, though this would be much more likely to produce the disease if the child's brain were in an overstrained condition.

The tendency for parents to send their children to school as soon as they have recovered from acute illnesses, is greatly to be deprecated.* After fevers, for instance, it takes some months before the brain recovers its former condition of nutrition and power. After severe blows on the head, or concussion of the brain, again, children should be allowed prolonged mental rest, or a tendency to epilepsy or other diseases may be developed.

Excessive study is a mistake, from every point of view. It defeats its own ends; the mind cannot assimilate beyond a certain rate, any more than can the digestive organs; and it

---

* The insistance by School-Board officers of an early return to school of children who have been seriously ill, is a real evil, which falls heavily on the poor.

makes study distasteful to children, and consequently encourages the shirking of tasks.

It is a mistake also, because it assumes that the *acquisition* of knowledge is everything, forgetting that the *organisation* of knowledge, for which time and thought are required, is the essentially important matter. " It is not the knowledge stored up as intellectual fat which is of value, but that which is turned into intellectual muscle." (Herbert Spencer.)

The folly of what is known as the " cram " system becomes evident in this connection. The knowledge imparted in such a way is speedily lost, while at the same time the brain is unfitted for healthful and spontaneous exercise in the future.

It is a mistake also, because, in the young, it interferes with the due development of the whole body. The increased circulation of blood in the brain implies diminished circulation through the limbs and other parts of the system. Even supposing that increased mental power *is* the result, the general physique necessary to make it available in the battle of life, is wanting; unless a man is "a good animal," one of the first requisites for success in life is absent. But increased mental power is not the result. The abnormally-rapid advance of any organ in respect of structure, involves premature arrest of its growth. A forced brain usually falls short, in the end, of the normal standard of size and power.

Many causes may, in badly-arranged schools, lead to the production of over-strain in children.

They may be classified as influences operating through the general health, home-lessons, bad arrangement of work, examinations, and punishments.

(1.) Very often the amount of work is not in itself excessive, but *the scholar's health is depreciated* by deficient exercise, impure air, deficient clothing, or insufficient or unsuitable food. These matters will be discussed in later chapters.

(2.) Not uncommonly the school-lessons are not excessive, but *home-lessons* are given which require prolonged attention, and leave too little time for meals or recreation. Parents can best judge as to whether home-lessons are doing harm, and and should at once communicate with the teacher, if any indications of over-pressure appear. In any case, home-lessons should be reduced to a minimum, should not require to be done in the evening, and should rather take the form of recapitulation of work done during the day than break into new ground.

(3.) *The School-work may be badly arranged.*—The most common fault under this head is too long lessons. The brain becomes fatigued when attention to one subject is prolonged. Much better results can be obtained in an hour's lesson by devoting five minutes in the middle of it to drill-exercises, than if the whole hour is devoted to mental work. Lessons should never exceed an hour in duration even for elder scholars, and three-quarters of an hour is preferable. Singing or drill-exercises for a few minutes in the interval arouse the nervous energies and facilitate subsequent attention to work.

Even during school-hours much can be done to diminish fatigue by *change of subjects*. Thus languages or history should alternate with mathematics, memory and reasoning being successively exercised. Then mechanical work, as writing or drawing, may follow, succeeded by object-lessons and experimental lectures. By some such succession as this the best results can be obtained with the least mental fatigue. In this connection, the proposed introduction of technical and industrial instruction into elementary schools is a most important step in the right direction, and will have invaluable influence on both the mental and physical training of children. The time devoted to manual instruction, while it is useful in itself as an introduction to industrial occupations, has an important bearing, which has already been discussed, on the due development of every part of the brain, and on the maintenance of that balance between different parts, upon which healthful and co-ordinated mental action depends.

(4) *Examinations* are chiefly sources of danger to older scholars, especially when they are of a competitive character, bringing into action the force of emulation. The mobile nervous system, and the somewhat greater preponderance of the emotional faculties in girls, render them peculiarly prone to suffer when subjected to competitive examinations.

We are not prepared to condemn examinations; it would be difficult or even impossible to discover an efficient substitute. If well conducted, an examination may be of great educative value. It finds out weak points, and shows how future efforts may be made more successful, while the anticipation of the examination guides and stimulates the scholar's efforts. The best results of a teacher's work, especially his personal influence on the training of mental or moral faculties, and the influence of an upright and consistent example, can, however, never be brought to the test of an examination.

Doubtless the best motive for studying a subject would be the interest it affords; but this cannot be aroused till the scholar enters the subject, and sometimes not even then; hence the necessity for some external definite motive.

Examinations at the best are but means to an end; they cease to be beneficial when they are made the object of the teacher's tuition, and they are most pernicious when undue strain is put on children for some weeks before the known date of an examination rather than a steady unwavering system of work throughout the year. Examinations, in order to be satisfactory, should review the work actually done by the scholar. The duty of the examiner is rather to find out how much the scholar knows, than to distress him by revealing his ignorance on obscure points. An examination of the former kind may be a healthful and encouraging stimulus, while one of the latter kind leaves only a sense of embarrassment and irritation in the scholar's mind, which weakens him for future efforts.

The occurrence of headaches, restlessness, irritability, and inability to fix the attention, are finger-posts showing over-work in preparation for examinations, and should receive early attention.

In 1872 the Massachusetts Board of Health enquired by circular of a number of physicians and teachers whether in their experience phthisis (consumption) was ever brought on by over-study. Of 191 replies, 146 were in the affirmative, and Dr. Bowditch, then Chairman of the Board, said: "I find almost invariably in patients predisposed to phthisis, that a prize gained or an examination concluded is the signal for entire decay of the physical powers, under the violent strain put previously on the mind, and with a total neglect of corresponding physical exercise." The fact that such a large proportion of answers were in the affirmative is not so conclusive as at first sight appears; for those doctors having definite cases to narrate would be much more likely to answer the circular than others whose experience was negative.

(5.) *Punishments* are a valuable means of bringing refractory children to reason; though the fear of them, when wielded by an unmerciful teacher, may lead nervous children to excessive and injurious efforts.

The advisability of corporal punishment is a somewhat vexed question. It is urged against it that it is hurtful and degrading to those who receive it, while it hardens the sensibilities of those who inflict it. The latter is certainly not true, if the punishment is moderate, and not inflicted under the influence of passion. As regards the former, most teachers assert that there are children so wayward and obstinate, that there is no way of controlling them except through fear of bodily pain. If bodily punishment is ever inflicted, it should be as a last resort, and at an hour-or-two's interval after the offence requiring it, in order that the punishment may not be vindictive, and that it may be quite clear to the delinquent that the teacher is simply the instrument of punishment which is the natural result of the offence.

Certain forms of corporal punishment should never be allowed. Boxing the ears or blows on the head are always dangerous, and so is the use of a hard inflexible stick.

It would appear that teachers are gradually finding that they can maintain discipline without any form of corporal punishment. In the city of New York it has been forbidden in the public schools, expulsion being substituted for it as a *dernier ressort*.

The giving of impositions requiring the keeping-in of the scholar for a prolonged period, and interfering with his meals and recreation, should seldom be had recourse to. The plan of having good and bad marks, which are subsequently reported to parents and made the subject of rewards, works much better than any form of corporal punishment.

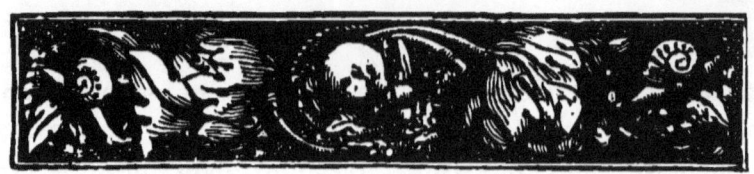

CHAPTER XI.

AGE AND SEX IN RELATION TO SCHOOL-WORK.

Duration of School-work at various Ages.—Statistics of Children attending School at various Ages.—Growth and Development in relation to School work.—Weight and Size of Children.—Chart of Growth of Children.—Sex in Education.—Character of Education in relation to Sex.

AGE has a most important bearing on the character, amount, and distribution of the work to be given to children. During the period of *childhood*, including up to the end of the 7th year, more rapid changes are being undergone than at any subsequent period of life. At 7 years old a child weighs about 6 times as much as at birth, and has half the stature, and from one-third to one-fourth of the weight of an adult. The less book-work the better, during this period. Education is not confined to schools. From the first moment of life education in the best sense commences, and makes rapid strides. The senses become trained, and the powers of observation are perhaps keener than at any subsequent period, while the mind is becoming stored with impressions which form the groundwork of subsequent mental life.

Much depends on the general training of a child during this period. His habits are being formed, and his after-progress in life is largely determined by the parental and other influences to which he is at this time subjected.

Various opinions are held as to the age at which attendance at school should begin. The following table gives the percentage at different ages, for the 4,412,148 children attending public elementary schools in England and Wales during the year 1885. (Report of Committee of Council on Education, 1885-6, p. 210.)

Age.	Per cent.	Age.	Per cent.
Under 3 years.	·20	8–9	11·95
3—4	2·89	9—10	11·74
4—5	6·58	10—11	11·45
5—6	10·00	11—12	10·11
6—7	11·40	12—13	7·81
7—8	11·77	13—14	3·21
		14 and over	·89

It will be seen from this table that 10 per cent. of the total number of scholars attending school are under 5 years of age, and that 31 per cent. are under 7 years of age. This strikingly shows that there is a marked tendency to crowd the work of school-education into the very early years of life, and it is therefore of the greater importance to consider what should be the nature of this education from a hygienic standpoint, in order that the danger which such early attendance implies, may be averted.

What education then may safely be given at such an age? We have already pointed out that in the early years of life the powers of observation are alone among the mental functions which are in active operation. To these, then, the instruction must be primarily addressed. If the mental activities of subsequent years are anticipated, and the reflective powers are prematurely stimulated, the result cannot be otherwise than disastrous to the mental and physical health of the child.

Undoubtedly the zeal of elementary school teachers has tended in the latter direction, and it is interesting to note that in the later forms of school laws, a sounder and more physiological method is being approached. The "merit grant" in infant-schools can now be obtained only on condition that simple lessons on objects, and on the phenomena of nature, and of common life (which appeal primarily to the senses and the powers of observation) are given, attended by appropriate and varied occupations. This is a valuable step in the right direction, and will require further extension, if future generations are to be saved from that stunted growth of the mind and body, which premature and excessive stimulation of the powers of reflection and memory cannot fail to produce.

The next period of life is that of *boyhood or girlhood*—extending from the 7th to the 14th year or from the appearance of the permanent teeth to puberty.

A child seven years old is unable to attend to any one subject beyond a limited time. According to Mr. Edwin Chadwick a pioneer in all sanitary and social reform, a single lesson between the ages of 5 and 7 should last only 15 minutes; between 7 and 10 about 20 minutes; from 10 to 12 about 25 minutes; 12 to 16 about 30 minutes. These limits are too restricted for the higher ages and for interesting subjects, but the principle involved is most important.

The amount of work should always be carefully graduated according to age. For children from 7 to 8 years old, work should not last longer than $2\frac{1}{2}$ to 3 hours a-day; from 8 to 10, from 3 to $3\frac{1}{2}$ hours; from 10 to 12, about 4 hours; from 12 to 15, between 5 and 6 hours; and from 15 to 18, never more than 8 hours, intervals being allowed for recreation.

Mr. Edwin Chadwick has maintained that under the "half-time" system, children make as good progress as if they attended school the whole day. Whether this is confirmed or not, there can be no question that the alternation of directed manual labour (see page 66), with shorter periods of study, would be attended with the greatest advantage to the mental and physical development of children.

If at the earlier ages more than 3 hours' work is required, the work becomes too exciting, and children become prematurely clever, which involves great risks and no genuine gain. Precocious children seldom realise the promise they gave.

It must be carefully remembered that during the period of school-life *growth and development* of every organ are, under natural conditions, rapidly proceeding, and that, while diligently cultivating the brain, the rest of the body must not be neglected. There is to some extent an antagonism between *growth* (*i.e.*, increase in size), and *development* (*i.e.*, increase in structure). The undue and premature elaboration of structure, as in mental precocity, involves a stoppage or diminution of growth, and ultimately a feebler brain. *We do not wish it to be inferred that brains should, so to speak, be allowed to lie fallow until their growth is completed, and then have their structure elaborated by mental education. This would be as impossible as it is undesirable. We only wish to state the

---

* For a very valuable detailed discussion of this and other matters bearing on the physiological aspect of education, see the article by Sir Crichton Browne, M.D., on "Education and the Nervous System," in Cassell's *Book of Health*. It is a pity that this Essay is not published separately for the use of teachers and others interested in the subject.

importance of not over-exciting the juvenile brain, and thus causing it to fall short of the size and power it would otherwise have attained. The difference has been well stated thus :—At 10 years old we may assume the brain to be a 10-carat brain. Push on education and make it rapidly the 24-carat brain it should become only with adult life, and the result will be that the total value obtained owing to the smaller amount of brain will be much less than if the forcing system had not been adopted.

The evil results of undue excitement of the brain during the period of growth are not confined to that organ. The brain has great influence over all other functions of the body. A fastidious appetite, imperfect digestion, or weak circulation, followed by retarded growth of body and general enfeeblement, are not uncommon results of hard study, when insufficient time is allowed for recreation and other purposes.

It would be well if every parent would at intervals of three months or even oftener have his children weighed and measured, keeping a record of the result.

Such information is easily obtained and would be of immense value in warning as to the insidious onset of disease, or a too rapid increase in stature. It is well known that when a boy is growing very rapidly his powers of mental application become greatly diminished. He is dull and apathetic, and perhaps lays himself open to undeserved censure, which might have been averted had the parent informed the teacher of the rapid growth and consequent necessity for diminution of work. Any increase in size beyond 2 to 3 inches a year involving undue strain on the system, or any sudden stoppage of growth (indicating perhaps the onset of consumption or other diseases, especially if accompanied by diminished weight) should excite apprehension and lead to medical supervision.

Stoppage of growth or of increase in weight might be due

(1) to insufficient food or clothing, the food being required to keep up the temperature of the body and no surplus being left for purposes of growth ; or (2) to excessive mental work and deficient exercise in the open air ; or (3) to the onset of some disease. In all cases it requires careful attention even when no other indications of disorder are present.*

Height and Weight of Children.—The following tables give valuable information respecting the height, weight, and rate of growth of boys and girls. They are taken from a most valuable paper by Dr. Bowditch, of Harvard University, on " The Growth of Children," in the 8th Annual Report of the Massachusetts Board of Health for 1877, and I have specially arranged them so as to compare boys of different classes, and boys with girls. For the figures contained in Table I., Dr. Bowditch is indebted to Mr. C. Roberts, of London. In each

---

* The following remarks of Mr. Sharpe, H.M. Inspector of Training Colleges, may be quoted as bearing on this point (Report of Committee of Council on Education, 1885-6, page 403):—" I should recommend to other colleges a practice, so far as I know, pursued by only one training college, viz , Westminster, the weighing of the students at regular intervals and recording the weights. At the beginning of the year 1885, all the students (over a hundred in number), with only three exceptions (all of them in their second year), increased steadily in weight. The annual inspection took place in the fifth month ; after the inspection it was found that only two of the second year's students had continued to increase in weight (one of whom had been steadily losing weight for three months and had begun to recover), and the average loss in weight per student during the few weeks preceding the examination was no less than 3lbs. The experienced vice-principal, Mr. Mansford, has no doubt that the loss of weight is solely attributable to the anxiety connected with the preparation and giving of lessons. This is the only form of over-pressure which is to be found in the male training colleges, and it would be difficult to find a healthier body of young men."

I may add that in the same college, when students have been found for two or three months to decrease in weight (the usual rule being a steady increase), I have been asked to examine into their physical condition. In several cases this has led to the early detection of disease, and in this way a break-down has been prevented.

TABLE I.

Average Height (in inches) and Weight (in pounds) of English Boys in Towns belonging to the Labouring Classes, compared with Children of Non-Labouring Classes belonging to Public Schools and Universities.

Age last Birthday	5	6	7	8	9	10	11	12	13	14	15	16	17	18	19	20	Total No. of Observations.
Average Height of Boys of the Non-Labouring Classes	—	—	46·10	47·66	50·30	52·65	53·93	55·90	58·30	60·27	63·00	65·34	66·91	67·38	67·74	68·09	5919
Average Height of Boys of Labouring Classes	41·15	43·18	45·15	46·81	48·82	50·28	51·83	53·02	54·24	56·37	59·81	63·45	65·50	66·00	66·50	67·00	10683
Average Growth—Non-Labouring	—	—	—	1·56	2·64	2·35	1·28	1·97	2·40	1·97	2·73	2·34	1·57	0·47	0·36	0·35	
Average Growth—Labouring	—	2·03	1·97	1·66	2·01	1·46	1·55	1·19	1·22	2·13	3·44	3·6;	2·05	0·50	0·50	0·50	
Average Weight—Non-Labouring	—	—	50·16	55·40	61·96	67·22	73·31	78·96	85·27	96·40	107·25	115·96	131·23	136·66	142·00	145·23	5361
Average Weight—Labouring	44·20	49·68	51·85	55·15	60·58	64·59	69·00	72·78	77·38	89·39	100·66	114·55	130·45	139·50	143·00	146·55	10871
Average Increase—Non-Labouring	—	—	—	6·24	5·56	5·26	6·09	5·65	6·31	11·13	10·85	8·71	15·97	4·75	5·32	3·23	
Average Increase—Labouring	—	5·48	2·21	3·26	5·43	4·01	4·41	3·78	4·60	12·01	11·27	13·89	15·90	9·05	3·50	·55	

TABLE II.

Average Height, Weight, and Growth of 13,691 Boys, and of 10,904 Girls in the Schools of Boston, Mass.—(Dr. Bowditch.)

Age last Birthday	5	6	7	8	9	10	11	12	13	14	15	16	17	18	Total No. of Observations.
Average Height of Boys	41·57	43·75	45·74	47·76	49·69	51·68	53·33	55·11	57·21	59·88	62·30	65·00	66·16	66·66	
,, ,, Girls	41·29	43·35	45·52	47·68	49·37	51·34	53·42	55·88	58·16	59·94	61·10	61·59	61·92	61·95	
Average Growth of Boys	—	2·18	1·99	2·02	1·93	1·99	1·65	1·78	2·10	2·67	2·42	2·70	1·16	0·50	
,, ,, Girls	—	2·06	2·17	2·06	1·79	1·97	2·08	2·46	2·28	1·78	1·16	0·49	0·33	0·03	
Average Weight of Boys	41·09	45·17	49·07	53·92	59·23	65·30	70·18	76·92	84·84	94·91	107·10	121·01	127·49	132·55	
,, ,, Girls	39·66	43·28	47·46	52·04	57·07	62·35	68·84	78·31	88·65	98·43	106·08	112·03	115·53	115·16	
Average Increase of Boys	—	4·08	3·90	4·85	5·31	6·07	4·88	6·74	7·92	10·07	12·19	13·91	6·48	5·06	
,, ,, Girls	—	3·62	4·18	4·58	5·03	5·28	6·49	9·47	10·34	9·78	7·65	5·95	3·50	0·63	
Number of Observations for Boys	848	1258	1419	1481	1437	1363	1293	1253	1160	908	636	359	192	84	13691
,, ,, ,, Girls	605	987	1199	1299	1149	1089	836	935	830	675	459	353	233	155	10904

table the heights are measured without shoes, and the weights in ordinary in-door clothing.

Many important particulars can be gathered from these tables. Thus the relationship which should hold between growth in height and increase in weight is easily calculated.

The ages at which growth is most rapid are easily seen. The greatest annual increase of height occurs for girls at 12, and for boys at 16 years. The greatest increase of weight for boys occurs at 16, and for girls at 13 years.

The influence of town life and labouring class is seen in the lower stature at all ages of children of this class. The most favoured class has a mean height 2 inches greater than the industrial class, the difference attaining a maximum of over 4 inches at 13 years of age.

Dr. Bowditch summarises his results as follows :—(1) During the first twelve years of life boys are from 1 to 2 inches taller than girls of the same age. (2) At about $12\frac{1}{2}$ years of age, girls begin to grow faster than boys, and during their 14th year are about one inch taller than boys of the same age. (3) At about $14\frac{1}{2}$ years boys again become the taller, girls having at this period very nearly completed their growth, while boys continue to grow rapidly till 19 years of age.

The same general results have been obtained in England, Mr. C. Roberts finding that girls of 13 years are as a rule taller and heavier than boys at the same age.

The bearing of the different rates of growth in the two sexes on the methods of healthy education will be discussed in the next paragraph.

The following chart has been copied by permission of Messrs. Macmillan from the "Life History Album," edited by F. Galton, F.R.S. It illustrates graphically the same facts as have been given in the preceding tables, and the observations,

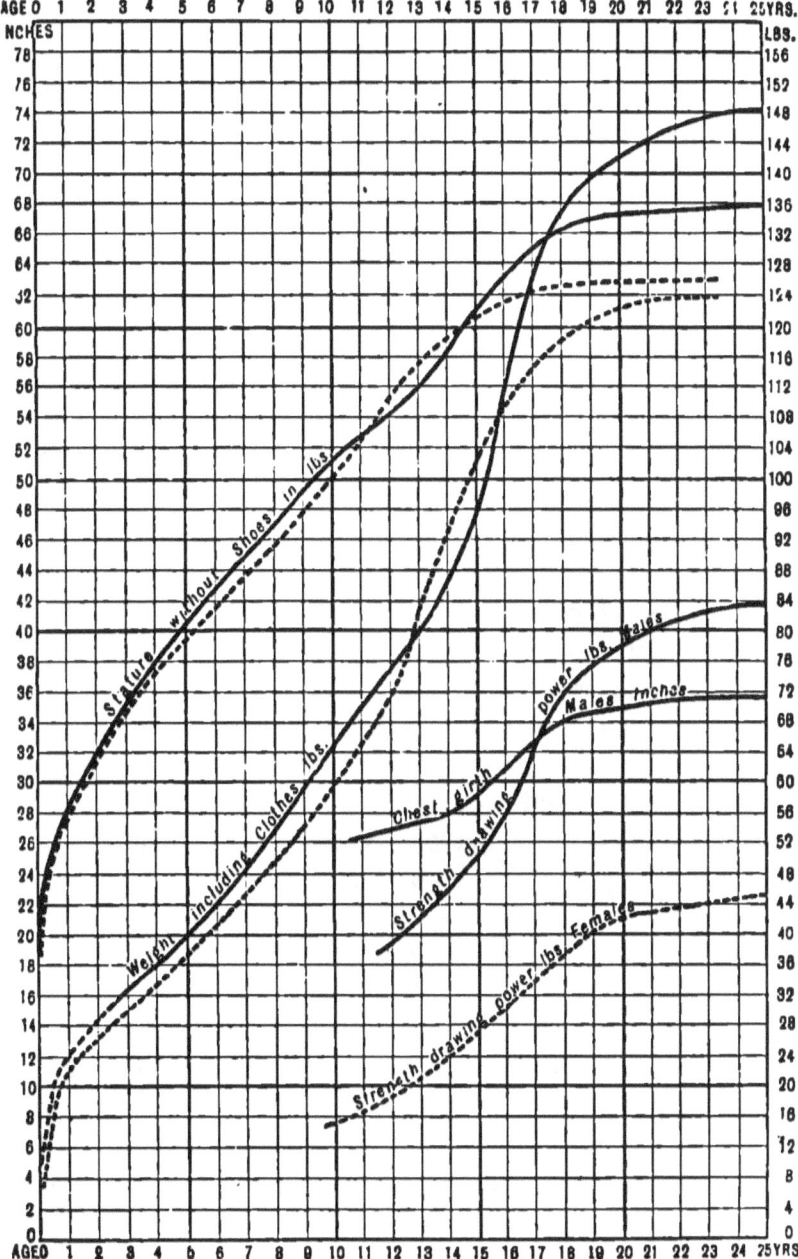

FIG. 18.—Chart showing average stature weight, chest girth, and strength of both sexes, from birth to 25 years of age, of the general population of the United Kingdom.
Males ——— Females ....
For "stature without shoes in *lbs.*," read *inches*.

although derived from a different source, support the same general conclusions.

Sex in Education.—Most of what has been already stated concerning the bearings of age on school-work applies equally to boys and girls. It is important to remember however that, as already stated, while growth of boys continues till manhood, girls concentrate a great deal of growth in a few years.

Owing to the relatively greater growth of girls from 12½ to 14½ or 15, it is particularly important that their height and weight should be watched during this period, and any over-strain from examinations or other source avoided. A stoppage of increase in weight or height should receive immediate attention, and even more important a continuance of growth in a girl who has ceased to become heavier may be one of the earliest indications of threatened consumption.

The period of puberty involves greater and more rapid changes in girls than in boys, and schooling requires to be carefully regulated at this period. Accompanying the changes in other organs, great changes must occur in the brain, new emotions and new phases of mental activity being developed. That the nervous system is unstable at this period is shown by the large amount of epilepsy which starts about puberty, and the still larger amount of hysteria. Insanity again is not uncommon after puberty, very rare before it.

The Massachusetts Board of Health in 1874 issued a circular asking teachers, physicians, &c., whether they found that puberty increased the liability to suffer from school attendance. Of 141 answers received, 120 were in the affirmative. It is probable that a carefully regulated school education is beneficial to girls of 14 to 17 rather than otherwise, and that the effects, which are sometimes ascribed to school-work, are more commonly due to defective exercise, late hours, and bad atmosphere, and the excitement of novels, or of a premature entry into society. An amount of mental work, which would be health'ul if followed by active and pleasant exercise, may be injurious when exercise is confined to a walk to and from school unaccompanied by any "play."

Undue devotion to music seems to have a specially exciting influence on some girls, and prolonged musical exercises are never desirable. Emulation in connection with examinations is much more likely to be injurious to girls than to boys.

At certain periods many physicians assert that school attendance should be temporarily suspended. We are not inclined to take this view in the majority of cases. Home lessons should be diminished, long walks or calisthenics should be stopped, and excitement should be avoided; but, as a rule, school attendance will do no harm.

Character of Education in relation to Sex.—Two opposite schools of thought have been vigorously advocated. It is the opinion of one that school education should be specially adapted to the peculiarities of each sex, while advocates of the other school strongly insist on equal and like education of the two sexes. Dr. Clarke, in his essay on *Sex in Education*, says : " None doubt the importance of age, acquirement, idiosyncrasy and probable career as factors in classification. Sex goes deeper than any of these." We are inclined to admit the justice of this, though laying a little more stress on the consideration that education should be adapted to the *individual* rather than to the *sex*. If this consideration be kept in mind, the absurdity of pressing on girls the study of higher mathematics, or the severer sciences, will be evident. Doubtless most girls are quite competent for these studies, if taken in moderation and with due consideration for the physical system, but the necessity for them is absent, and the time would be much better spent in developing a robust physical frame, competent for the practical functions of life. The painter who used up all his colours for his background, and left none for the portrait, is an apt illustration of the over-educated school-girl, lacking in practical knowledge and physique.

The female temperament is more nervous and excitable than the male, and the opportunities for counteracting the effects of mental work by vigorous muscular exertion are fewer. The evils of over-strain occur chiefly in girls between 13 and 18, and much danger would be averted if the considerations respecting exercise, to be advanced in the next chapter, were acted on in their case.

CHAPTER XII.

MUSCULAR EXERCISE AND RECREATION.

Analogy between Mental and Muscular Exercise.—Influence of Exercise on the System.—Influence on the Brain.—Excessive Exercise.—Deficient Exercise.—Rules for Exercise.—Forms of Exercise—Gymnastics.—Calisthenics.

THE voluntary muscles of the body contain in their substance about one-fourth of the whole volume of blood, and, even during their rest, important heat-producing and other functions are carried on in them, though these are rendered much more active by exercise.

Much of what has been said concerning brain exercise applies equally to the muscles. Just as the powers of memory, observation, judgment, speech, &c., increase by careful cultivation, so does muscular power. The brain is temporarily exhausted by fatigue, and so are the muscles; it may be permanently injured by excessive and prolonged exertions, and so likewise may the muscles, especially the heart-muscle.

Muscular exercise is important during school-life, because of its influence (1) on the general health, and (2) on the brain.

(1.) In consequence of the increased size and strength of the muscles produced by systematic exercise, they respond more easily to impulses of the will. The action of the lungs is increased, and consequently more pure air is inhaled, and more impurities are got rid of, while the actual capacity of the lungs, as indicated by the girth of the chest, becomes increased by well regulated exercise. In this way a flat-chested condition may be averted, and a tendency to consumption may be eradicated. The action of the skin is increased, and thus another means of elimination of impurities is set at work. The circulation is improved and rendered more uniform, and the production of heat is increased during exercise, in consequence of which cold feet and chilblains are avoided.

The following tables from Maclaren's " Physical Education " strikingly illustrate the valuable results obtainable from systematic gymnastic exercises.

The first table shows the effect of $7\frac{1}{2}$ months' training of men varying in age from 19 to 28, the average age being 24, the men having been irregularly selected.

	Weight.	Chest girth.	Girth of fore-arm.	Girth of upper arm
	lbs.	in.	in.	in.
The smallest Gain ...	5	1	$\frac{1}{4}$	$\frac{1}{4}$
The largest Gain ...	16	5	$1\frac{1}{4}$	$1\frac{3}{4}$
The average Gain ...	10	$2\frac{7}{8}$	$\frac{3}{4}$	$1\frac{3}{4}$

The second table shows the effect on two articled pupils, aged 16 and 20, of a year's steady practice in gymnastic exercises.

MUSCULAR EXERCISE AND RECREATION. 85

In the year's work the increase was—

	Height.	Weight.	Chest.	Fore-Arm.	Upper Arm.
	in.	lbs.	in.	in.	in.
With the younger	2	21	5	2	2
With the elder	$\frac{3}{8}$	$8\frac{1}{2}$	6	$1\frac{1}{4}$	$1\frac{1}{2}$

(2.) During the period of school-life the brain and muscles are both undergoing growth and development. They cannot be separated from one another, being intimately in communication by means of nerves. There is a motor part of the brain corresponding to the muscles, in which are stored ideas of weight, distance, resistance, the result of muscular contractions; and from which are carried the voluntary impulses which result in muscular exercise. This extensive region of the brain is in intimate communication with all the other regions of the brain, and at the same time it can attain its full vigour only when the whole muscular system is in a well developed and healthy condition. It is a well-known fact that each nervous centre requires external stimuli to develop its potential power. If a number of chickens are hatched on a carpet they will run about and never attempt to scratch until a little gravel is scattered on it. In two cases the congenital absence of the left hand and atrophy of the left arm was found after death to be associated with an atrophied condition of the convolution of the brain, in which movements of the hand are stated by Ferrier to be produced. But where death has occurred some years after amputation of the limb of an adult, no alteration in the corresponding part of the brain has been found. Hence the greater importance of exercise before twenty than after that age. The blindness of the fishes living in the dark caves of Kentucky is another instance of atrophy of a disused organ, and of the corresponding part of the brain.

The above considerations render it evident that the development of a considerable portion of the brain is dependent on muscular exercise, and the non-recognition of this principle has been saved from calamitous results in the past, only by the instinctive revelling of children in movements of every kind.

Excessive muscular exercise produces fatigue. If proper intervals of rest are not allowed this may end in serious disease, though such a result chiefly occurs when, as in clerks, a small group of muscles is over-worked, and writer's palsy is produced.

Violent over-exertion, such as occurs in competitive running or rowing, is very pernicious. The "broken winded" condition in horses is produced in a similar way. Occasionally the heart becomes dilated, or spitting of blood is produced. Competitive exercises always require careful and graduated preparation, and no boy should be allowed to join in them without previous medical examination.

We do not wish our sons to become as muscular as Hercules from over-muscular development, nor to be nervous and excitable and under-grown from the opposite condition, but to have their muscular and nervous systems healthy and in proper co-ordination. There is no necessary antagonism between mental culture and athleticism, except when the latter is indulged to excess.

The danger of excessive exercise is greatest during the period of most rapid growth between the ages of 15 and 17. Excessive muscular exercise may then interfere with growth, though deficient exercise is to be deprecated. Sometimes a boy at school grows from 6 to 8 inches in a year, and it is evident that all his strength is being expended in this direction.

Deficient exercise during school-life is much commoner

than excessive exercise, especially in girls. The general health is consequently impaired, digestion is enfeebled, the circulation becomes unequal, and nervous irritability and sleeplessness often supervene. The tendency to lung diseases, especially consumption, is greatly increased. The effects on the figure are lamentable. Drooping shoulders, a flat chest, stooping gait, and lateral curvature of the spine are natural consequences of flabby muscles destitute of tone. In girls the tendency to spinal curvature is increased by the tight imprisonment of the trunk in corsets which effectually prevent exercise of the trunk muscles. For girls who are growing rapidly, the use of Liebreich's chair, which is adapted to the curves of the spinal column, and gives complete rest to the spine, is very valuable. (Fig. 19). Reading or other work can be continued while resting in the chair. The alternation of such rest, with exercises specially adapted to strengthen the muscles of the back and shoulders, is most important in all cases where there is a tendency to spinal curvature, or drooping shoulders, or a forward stoop.

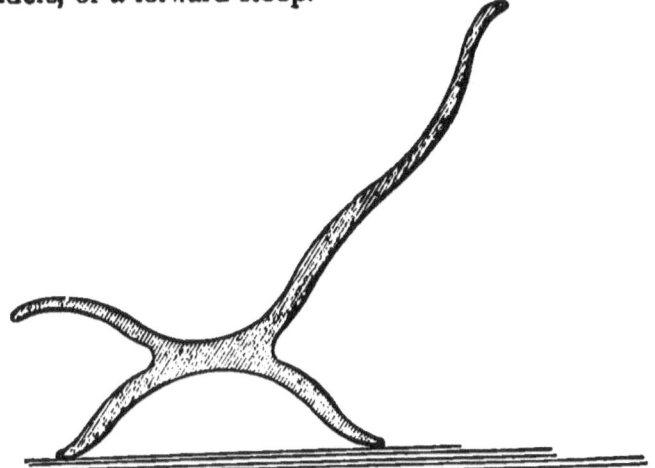

FIG. 19.—Chair giving complete spinal support.

In taking exercise the *following rules* should be regarded. The clothing should allow free play of the limbs, and expansion of the chest, flannel being always worn next the skin. Chill, which is so often produced by sitting in a draught after perspiration, must be carefully avoided. The exercise must be systematic and regular, and never sudden and violent, and the amount of exercise must be regulated by individual fitness. Every part of the body must be exercised. Exercise must not be taken directly after meals.

It should as far as possible be taken in the open air. The fact that the amount of air inspired during exercise is greatly increased serves to emphasise this rule, and explains why the benefit of girls' calisthenics is greatly diminished by their being commonly taken indoors.

Forms of Exercise.—If there is one point more important than another it is that exercise should be as varied as possible. The spontaneous activity of children is more conducive to general strength and healthy brain-growth than any formal gymnastics. The latter can never form a complete substitute for games. The movements are more rigid, and less varied, and consequently sooner produce fatigue, and the competition which serves for a stimulus in gymnastics is a very poor substitute for the enjoyment accompanying varied play. The enjoyable mental excitement of games acts as a stimulant and tonic to the heart, accelerating the circulation and helping all the bodily functions.

The more purely recreative physical exercise is, the greater the relief from school-work. The tendency to provide play-grounds of insufficient size is, in this connection, very deplorable, though, when this is unavoidable, gymnastics should be resorted to.

Running, leaping, rowing, swimming, cricket, rackets, tennis, &c., all have their place, and are deservedly popular. Boating should be restricted to those who can swim. Football scrimmages should not be allowed, and the ball should never be taken in the hands. A belt should never be allowed round the waist, being one of the commonest causes of rupture.

Singing, speaking, and reading aloud are forms of muscular exercise which might with advantage be more systematically adopted. They are most valuable in strengthening the throat and lungs, and rendering them less prone to disease.

Gymnastics were carefully studied in ancient times, the Greeks having a perfect system, which was adopted by the Romans to a certain extent, though not in its best aspects, and among them was confined to the military class and athletes. The best modern system is Ling's, or the Swedish system, which is founded on anatomical data, and does not seek merely muscular development, but a general improvement of circulation and nerve power, all the parts being brought into balanced action.

Gymnastic exercises should be adapted to the age and physical constitution of each pupil. Much injury may be done by making all the members of a class go through the same exercises. Up to the age of 15 or 16 such light gymnastic exercises as are described and illustrated in "Sound Bodies for our Boys and Girls," by W. Blaikie, if carried out under the superintendence of a skilled teacher, are amply sufficient, and obviate the necessity for any complicated apparatus. After this age a more advanced course of gymnastic exercises may be the means of laying the foundation of permanent health and strength.

Military drill is a useful addition to school routine. It serves not only to teach order and promptitude of obedience, but is a valuable means of exercise.

Exercise for Girls in the form of gymnastics, or the schoolgirls' gymnastics, known as calisthenics, is even more important than for boys, inasmuch as, especially in towns, there are for them fewer opportunities of play, and they suffer from improper modes of dressing.

The only advantage calisthenics presents over play is that it ensures an equal and regular exercise of muscles.

It is important, however, that it should be made interesting, otherwise much of the benefit is lost. By the use of dumb-bells (which should not exceed 2 to 4 lbs. for girls), elastic bands with handles, &c., many varied exercises can be performed.

Girls suffer much more on account of deficient recreation than boys. The formal boarding-school walk on *fine* days is but a travesty on the exercise required, and has little effect in stimulating the circulation, or refreshing the mind. A recess of half an hour should be allowed in the middle of each morning's school-work, during which every girl should be obliged to go out and play in fine weather, or assemble for calisthenics in wet weather. It should be made impossible to think of work during this half-hour.

CHAPTER XIII.

Rest and Sleep.

Law of Rest and Action.—Partial Rest.—Complete Rest.—Duration of Sleep.—Rules respecting Sleep.—School Dormitories.

LIFE is made up of alternations of rest and action. Exercise of any organ of the body is followed by a necessary period of repose, during which effete matters are removed by the blood, and flesh nutritive material is supplied by the same fluid.

The only apparent exceptions are the heart and lungs, and these in reality obey the universal law, the only difference being that their rest is frequent and momentary, while that of other organs is at greater intervals and of longer duration.

The heart, for instance, contracts about once every second, but in the intervals of each contraction it rests $\frac{8}{11}$ of a second, or over 13 hours in the day.

The necessity for rest can be easily proved in the case of the sense of taste. If salt be kept in the mouth for a considerable time, the power of tasting it disappears, and returns in its original strength only after several hours. The temporary deafness from the noise of machinery, and the fact that after looking at a given colour for some time, only its complementary colour is visible, are other instances of the same law.

Rest may be partial or general.

Partial rest is obtained by change of occupation, bringing into play the activity of other organs.

The importance of varying school-work at frequent intervals, thus exercising different parts of the brain, has been already discussed (see page 66). Similarly in the last chapter we have emphasized the importance of recreative muscular exercise. By these two means, undue pressure of school-work may nearly always be prevented.

Sleep is the only form of complete and general rest. During sleep a diminished amount of blood flows through the brain, and the functional activity of its higher centres is abrogated. If a boy or girl eats and sleeps well, it can scarce be that his brain is over-worked. It is a mistake, however, to suppose that the evils of excessive mental work can be entirely compensated by prolonging sleep. The mental work must be diminished, and more time must also be allowed for recreation.

The average amount of sleep required at—

4 years old is		12 hours.	
7	,,	11	,,
9	,,	$10\frac{1}{2}$	,,
12-14	,,	9-10	,,
14-21	,,	9	,,

Children under 14 should be allowed a little more sleep in winter than in summer, and when growing very fast. Punctuality in the time of sleep is of great importance, owing to the habit acquired. Great drowsiness or wakefulness in children should always be looked into. The night screamings to which some children are liable may indicate overwork at school, but generally they occur apart from school-work in children of a very nervous temperament.

The regulation of children's sleep is a matter which chiefly lies with parents, and they may greatly help the school-teacher by attention to it. It is unfortunate that growing boys and girls are, especially in winter, so frequently taken to concerts or other evening meetings. No wonder that they appear next morning at school with dark rings about their eyes, and generally incapacitated for mental application.

The importance of sleeping in a pure atmosphere, and of having, during winter, a flannel jacket or other warm covering to the arms and shoulders, need only be referred to.

School Dormitories should never be used during the day for study or other purposes, as thus the atmosphere is rendered impure, and irregular habits are induced. The windows should be kept widely open during the day in order to ensure a thorough and prolonged sweep of fresh air through the rooms. Large and airy bedrooms are very desirable, as thus the rooms can be more thoroughly ventilated and the pupils better supervised.

The same rules for ventilation and warming apply as in the case of the school-rooms. It is obvious that inasmuch as the pupil passes at least one-third of each day in his bedroom, its atmosphere should be as pure as possible. Even with the best means of ventilation this cannot be secured, unless a sufficient cubic space is allowed for each pupil. The Government insists on 300 cubic feet for each pauper in our workhouses. Surely, at least this amount might be allowed in boarding-schools; whereas beds are frequently placed almost, or quite, in contact, and such overcrowding occurs as, if it happened in a common lodging-house, would lead to the prosecution of the landlord. We have seen (page 27) that not less than 1500 cubic feet of fresh air are required by each pupil per hour. But if the air is changed more than three or four times per hour, violent draughts are produced. It follows, therefore, that from 375 to 500 cubic feet of space should be allowed for each scholar in the bedroom, and preferably the latter amount. Masters will assert that the ventilating arrangements they have introduced obviate the necessity for this amount of space. This is nearly always inaccurate; and even if it were theoretically true, children (as well as their seniors) will close up any orifice from which an unpleasant draught is perceptible. Dr. Dukes, the Physician to Rugby School, urges that taking a school-bed at 3 by 6 feet, the superficial area of the bedroom should be 6 by 12 feet per pupil, and the room 12 feet high. This gives 864 cubic feet per head, which, allowing for the air displaced by the furniture of the room and the boy himself, leaves about 800 cubic feet per head. The poor health and pale appearance of children at boarding-schools are much oftener due to crowded bedrooms, than to insufficient or inferior food, or to overwork.

Each pupil should have his own towel and brush and comb. The interchange of these frequently leads to the spread of ringworm, or of contagious affections of the eye.

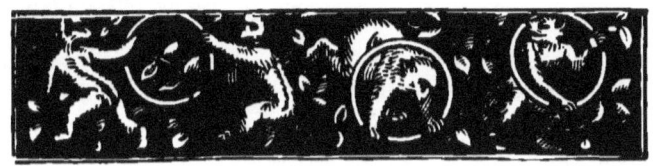

CHAPTER XIV.

CHILDREN'S DIET.

Quantity and Quality of Food.—Food required for Growth.—Relation of Food to Work.—Frequency of Under-feeding.—Amount of Food Required.

The diet of children should be generous and abundant.

There is no danger of giving too much food, if none but simple and wholesome dishes are allowed. After 40 it may be broadly said that the chief danger in regard to diet is of over-feeding, under 20 of under-feeding. It must be remembered that during youth, and up to the age of 25, physiological processes are much more active than at a later period; freer exercise is usually taken, and, in addition, food is required not only to supply force for carrying on the functions of the body, but also for purposes of growth. Children have to make new tissues as well as to keep in repair those already established. Also as their bodies expose more surface, in proportion to size, than adults, they require a proportionately larger amount of food to compensate for loss of heat.

It is only after waste of tissues and heat loss have been provided for, that any surplus of nutriment goes to the further growth of the body. Given that the food supply is scanty, one of two things must happen: growth will be impeded, and children will be stunted specimens of humanity; or some of the organs of the body, as the brain, or muscles, or bone, will suffer in functional activity, and may eventually become the actual seat of disease.

The younger an animal, the more easily is it starved; and the more actively growing are its organs, the more seriously injured by starvation; and the same applies to human beings.

Apart from the food required for growth and development, the close relationship between food and work must not be forgotten in the case of children as well as of the adult. Work can no more be done by a child without food than by a steam-engine without fuel. The more brain-work a child does, the more food he uses up. It is a great fallacy to suppose that food is less necessary for the brain-worker than for the navvy. Each metabolises (roughly speaking—oxidises) a large amount of combustible material, which must be supplied by food. The navvy, however, commonly acquires his combustible material with greater ease than the brain-worker, owing to his better digestion.

Hence the importance of not allowing half-starved children to be unduly burdened with mental work is evident. Even though they may with an effort succeed in their studies, it is at the expense of a diminutive stature and feeble muscles. It is to be hoped that the practice of giving penny dinners to children of Board Schools in poorer districts may extend. A still better plan would be to give them a mug of milk and slice of bread before the morning's work begins.

It is unhappily the case that the children even of wealthy people are frequently underfed. A certain amount is apportioned at each meal, and a lecture on the evils of greediness follows a request for more. We hold that a healthy child's appetite is the best guide as to the amount of food required, if only the food is plain and wholesome. He might surfeit himself with rich pastry, or cakes, but hardly with porridge and milk.

The danger of under-feeding is especially great among girls, a good appetite being not uncommonly regarded by them as something to be ashamed of. Girls between the ages of 14 and 20 often suffer from a species of chronic starvation, having got into the habit of relying on bread and butter and puddings, to the almost complete exclusion of meat, or other nitrogenous food. Much weakness and ill-health in after life are ascribable to this cause.

According to Dr. De Chaumont (Conference on School Hygiene at Health Exhibition), for a child weighing 100lbs. (who would probably be 15 years old, see chart, page 79), about 3 ozs. of albuminate (flesh-producing) food, $2\frac{1}{2}$ ozs. of fat, 12 ozs. of carbohydrates (starch and sugar), and about $\frac{3}{4}$ oz. of mineral matter are required per diem. In order to obtain the above amount of albuminate material, 6 ozs. of meat would be required, unless cheese, legumens (beans, peas, &c.), or milk are freely taken. It may be convenient to remember that bread contains about 8 per cent. albuminates (and 50 per cent. starch), meat 15 per cent. albuminates, cheese over 30 per cent. and peas and beans generally 22 per cent. Most dietaries contain abundance of starch and sugar, but are deficient in fat. This deficiency is a most important matter. If children will not eat the fat of meat, then dripping, butter, and suet puddings are useful.

Children's diet should be varied and palatable. The intervals between meals should be regular and not too long. The food should not be allowed to be bolted, but carefully chewed. Milk should form an important part of all children's diet. Alcohol should not be given in any form, unless under medical responsibility. The teeth should be carefully supervised; overcrowding of the permanent teeth should be prevented by the dentist's aid, and cavities should receive early attention.

H

The *water* supplied at school should be pure, and absolutely above suspicion. Impurities may be due to its being derived from an impure source, as a shallow well, or to impurities acquired in transit through the pipes, or to the cistern allowing contamination of the water, either through its being uncovered, or having its waste-pipe connected with some part of the drainage system. The filter should be frequently cleansed, or it may do more harm than good.

CHAPTER XV.

CHILDREN'S DRESS.

Amount of Clothing required.—Relation of Clothing to Food.—The Hardening Process.— Distribution of Clothing.—Rules respecting Clothing.

A CERTAIN temperature of the surface of the body (about 98·5 Fahr.) is necessary for the maintenance of health, and from this it never varies more than 18. This temperature is the result of the chemical processes going on in the body, the fuel for which is supplied by the food taken. Food being deficient, the body-temperature would necessarily fall, if there were no reserve of combustible material stored up in the tissues.

It is evident that heat may be economised, and thus within certain limits the amount of food required may be diminished by preventing some of the loss of heat from the body. About 80 to 90 per cent. of this loss being by the skin, clothing plays an important part in preventing loss of heat.

Clothing should prevent as far as possible radiation and con duction of heat, but not evaporation of the perspiration. The material which is in these respects best, both for summer and winter wear is wool, which should always be worn next the skin; the thickness, and not the material, being altered according to the external temperature.

The amount of clothing for children should be sufficient to prevent any sensation of cold. Excessive clothing may make children tender by increasing the tendency to catch cold, owing to its exciting perspiration, and to the fact that the extra clothing is often thrown off at irregular intervals. The effect of wearing a thick scarf round the neck is a well-known instance of this.

A deficient amount of clothing is even more dangerous. The attempt is commonly made to "harden" children to bear exposure to cold with bare arms and legs. The consequences of this hardening theory are most calamitous; not a few children are hardened out of the world, and those who survive suffer permanently, either in growth or constitution. The dwarfishness of Laplanders and Esquimaux is an illustration of this principle. Children produce heat less freely, and lose it more quickly, than adults, hence the great mortality of children in cold climates during the winter months.

Liebig first clearly explained the importance of clothing, saying: "Our clothing is, in reference to the temperature of the body, merely an equivalent for a certain amount of food." It will be easily understood, therefore, how deficient clothing, like deficient food, may produce stunted growth, or lay the foundation for disease, or bring latent disease into activity.

Children's clothing should be of such a character that the warmth is *uniformly distributed*. No extra amount of chest protection will prevent bronchitis or pneumonia, if the legs and feet are cold. The adoption of leggings and sleeves for young children should always be insisted on. *Thin boots* are especially objectionable. There is a great sympathy between the feet and the respiratory tract. Chest affections are frequently due to cold and damp feet. The boots should be thick enough to keep the feet dry and warm. It is advisable, in some cases, especially, for girls to bring a dry pair of stockings to school.

Damp garments should be laid aside at once on reaching home, and the teacher should never allow a scholar to remain in school with wet clothes.

The practice of wearing thicker outside garments while in the warm school-room is very objectionable. The skin becomes relaxed and perspiration occurs, and it only requires the subsequent exposure on the journey home to ensure a severe catarrh.

The clothing should not be changed according to the calendar, but according to the state of the weather.

The wearing of summer-clothing late into autumn, and the assuming of light outer-garments and under-clothing as soon as a fine day in spring appears, are very dangerous for children.

Moist cold is a good conductor of heat, and the damp chilliness of an early November requires as warm and thick clothing as the dry, clear cold of January.

Tight clothing of any kind should be avoided. It interferes with free movement and so prevents proper exercise.

Tight corsets are particularly objectionable, and belts round the waist. Tight sleeves and skirts prevent free movements of the limbs. Stockings should be supported by suspenders and not by garters. Tight boots destroy the natural elasticity of the movements, besides interfering with the circulation and thus causing cold feet. High-heeled boots produce an uncertain and ungraceful gait in girls; they throw the weight of the body on the front part of the feet, disturbing its balance, and tending to produce spinal curvature. The soles of shoes should be broader than the feet, the heels low and broad, and the soles should be thick enough to keep out all damp.

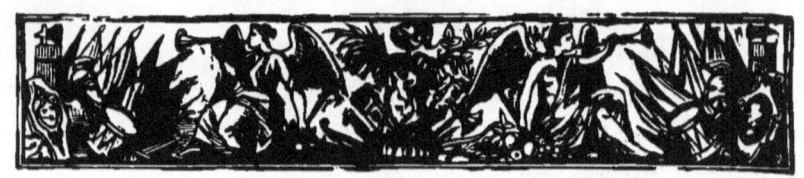

CHAPTER XVI.

BATHS AND BATHING.

Necessity for Cleanliness.—School Baths and Swimming.

IN previous chapters, the use of food and clothing in preventing loss of heat and maintaining a uniform temperature has been briefly discussed. In this chapter we wish briefly to impress the fact that the skin, by the proper use of water, may be brought into such a robust condition that the sudden alternations of temperature to which children are necessarily exposed, become comparatively free from danger.

No school education is complete which does not teach children the necessity for a clean skin. A dirty condition of the person strongly favours the incidence of infectious disease, as well as helps to produce that unpleasant odour which commonly belongs to the air of a school-room full of scholars.

The disuse of soap and cold water to the skin renders the cutaneous blood-vessels deficient in tone, and thus favours the production of chills. Where morning cold baths are not well borne by children, sponging with a wet towel, followed by friction with a dry rough towel, forms a good substitute.

It is impossible, even if it were desirable, always to keep children in warm rooms. They play about in cold corridors, or other places exposed to cold currents of air, and if their skin is lacking in tone, a sore throat or bronchitis may be the result.

School bathing is very desirable, though arrangements are seldom made for it. Schools containing several hundred boys can hardly be regarded as complete unless they possess a swimming-bath of their own, or one in some way open to them. Many unfortunate accidents would be prevented, and much gain to the health and happiness of children would result, if they were taught to swim. A boy accustomed to plunge into cold water (*i.e.* at 50° to 60°, not 32°), is much less likely to suffer from alternations of temperature than other children, and, if by chance he should get wet through, is less liable to be chilled or laid up by fever.

Swimming combines the advantages of bathing and exercise. A plunge into running water is more liable to produce cramp, or dangerous chilling of vital organs, than into the water of a swimming bath, as, in the former case, the water around the swimmer is constantly being changed, and so a greater abstraction of heat from the body occurs.

School bathing should always be under strict supervision. Children should not be allowed to loiter in undressing; they should never be allowed to remain in the water until chattering of teeth, or blueness of lips or nails is produced; and the bath should not be taken within two hours of a meal.

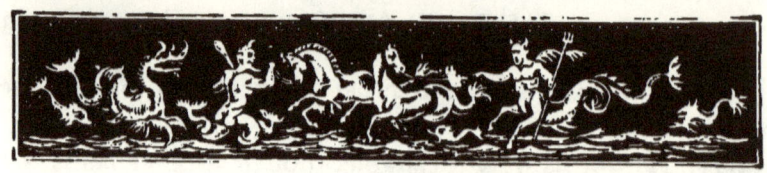

CHAPTER XVII.

EYESIGHT IN RELATION TO SCHOOL LIFE.

Structure of the Eye.—Causation of Long and Short Sight.—Use of Eyes for near Objects.—Inadequate Light.—Badly-printed Books. —Fine Needlework.—Influence of General Health on Eyesight.

IN order to understand the influence of school-life on eyesight the following facts relating to the structure of the eye are important.

The eye is enveloped throughout the greater part of its circumference by a dense white coat (the sclerotic), the transparent and more convex cornea enveloping the smaller moiety in front. (Fig. 20). Inside the sclerotic is a black vascular layer (the choroid), which serves to absorb excessive rays of light, and within this is spread out the delicate meshwork of the retina, which receives impressions of light and conveys them to the brain. The interior of the eyeball is occupied by a transparent gelatinous material in its posterior part, and a watery material in front, between which lies the delicate lens of the eye, which is capable of being altered in shape by the action of minute ciliary muscles. (3, Fig. 20).

In the normal eye, rays of light coming from a distance (*i.e.*, practically parallel rays) are refracted by the passive lens and media of the eye, and brought to a focus at the most sensitive part of the retina, without any muscular effort. Thus, vision of distant objects represents rest for the eyes, and exertion of its muscles comes into play only for near vision.

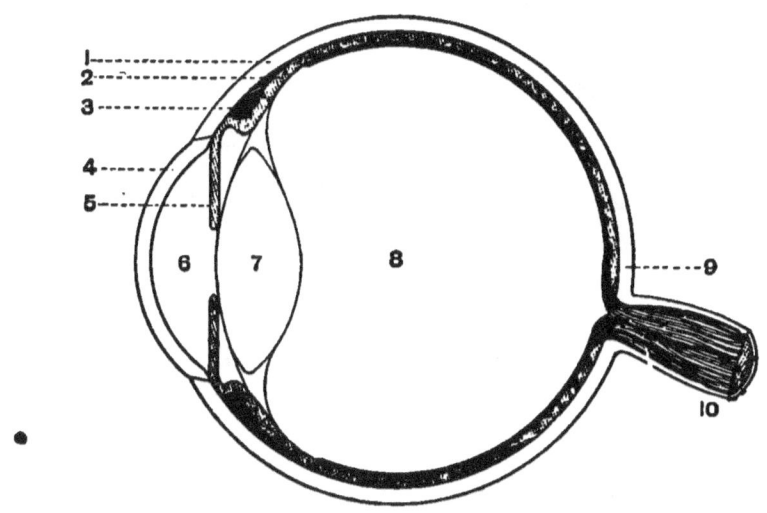

FIG. 20—Vertical section of the eyeball.
1, Sclerotic; 2, choroid; 3, ciliary muscle; 4 cornea; 5, iris; 6, aqueous humour; 7, lens; 8, vitreous humour; 9, retina; 10, optic nerve.

The divergent rays of light from a near object are brought to a focus on the retina by the action of the ciliary muscle, which renders the lens more convex, and thus capable of refracting the light more powerfully. The effect of an increased convexity of lens in bringing divergent rays of light sooner to a focus is shown in Fig. 21. If for any distance under 20ft. the eye were not able thus to accommodate its condition, a blurred and incomplete image would be formed on the retina.

A child with normal eyes ought to be able to read this page, in a good light at the distance of 40 inches, and at all intervening distances down to 4 inches. Any child who cannot

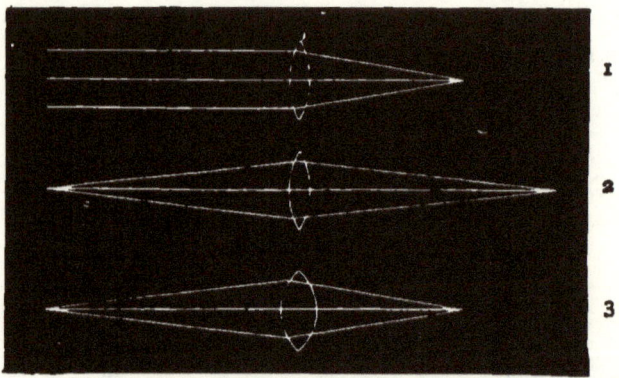

FIG. 21.—Diagram showing effect of a biconvex lens on rays of light. 1, Focus of parallel rays ; 2, focus of divergent rays ; 3, focus of divergent rays brought nearer by more convex lens.

read it as far as 15 inches off should have his eyes examined by a competent eye-surgeon. A rough test may be also made by means of the following letters :—The Z should be distinguishable at a distance of 50 feet, D at a distance of 40 feet, Y at 25 feet, H at 20 feet, and L at 10 feet.

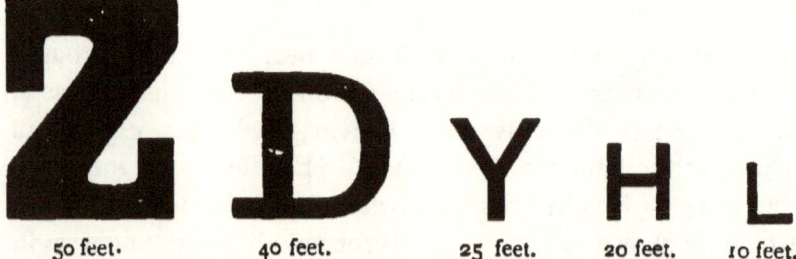

Three chief defects of vision occur in children ; in the first, the rays of light are brought to a focus behind the retina (hypermetropia); in the second, the rays of light are brought to a focus in front of the retina (myopia); and in the third, the different axes of the eyes do not bring rays of light to a focus at the same point (astigmatism).

Hypermetropia or *Long-sight*, in which the eye is shorter from behind forwards than usual, is really in a moderate degree a normal condition in childhood, but if present in a high degree represents an arrest of development. Parallel rays of light (*i.e.*, those from a distance) are brought to a focus behind the retina. (Fig. 22.) Thus, when the eye is at rest there is not

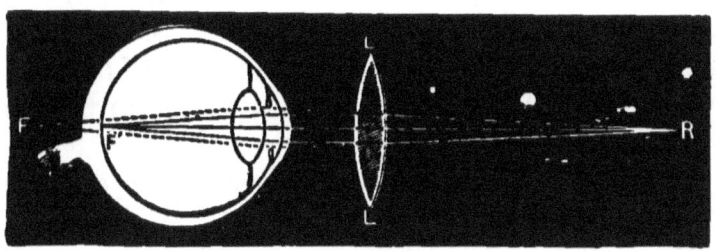

FIG 22.—Sec ion of hypermetropic eye.
R, the origin of divergent rays of light; F, the focus beyond the eyeball; LL, convex glasses to be worn by hypermetrope; F' the focus of rays of light on retina, showing influence of L.

distinct vision even of distant objects for the long-sighted. The ciliary muscles must always act and accommodate the eye, and in moderate degrees they succeed in concealing the condition. It is evident, however, that this constant strain on the muscles, during the waking hours, must be injurious; and during the use of the eye for near vision, as in reading or needlework, the strain on the ciliary muscles becomes still greater. Consequently, congestion and redness, with watering of the eyes, result.

The lids tend to stick together in the morning, owing to increased secretion. If close work is insisted on, in severe cases dizziness and total inability to distinguish letters are produced, and, in some cases, nausea, or even vomiting. The child is worse in the morning than the evening, as his ciliary muscles have to adjust themselves to the strain imposed on them. Mistakes are frequently made, and the child is often thought to be idle. In this, as in other abnormal conditions of the eye, it is very common for the child to have been repeatedly punished by his teachers for supposed obstinacy or stupidity.

Long-sight is often confused with short-sight, because, in the former, as in the latter, the child gradually holds his book nearer and nearer to his eyes. This is because spasm of the ciliary muscle (causing accommodation beyond the necessities of the case) is produced by the efforts to see small objects at moderate distances, and because the large size of the image of the print obtained by holding the book nearer partially compensates for its imperfect definition.

In the effort at accommodating long-sighted eyes for near and small objects, those external muscles of the eyeballs which turn them in towards the nose, are brought into excessive action. A convergent squint may be thus produced, at first occasional, afterwards becoming constant, and one eye being usually worse than the other. The squint is worse when the child is tired or ill, but any squint in a child 4 to 7 years old should receive immediate attention.

Myopia or *Short-sight* is the exact opposite of the last condition, the eye from before backwards being too long, so that rays of light from a distance are brought to a focus in front of the retina. In order that they may be focussed on the retina, the affected child finds it necessary to hold objects near his eye, thus making the rays of light more divergent.

Myopia is distinguished from hypermetropia by the fact that distant vision is improved by a concave lens, and by the fact that the smallest type can be read easily, provided it be held closely to the eyes.

The fact of a person seeing equally as well, at a distance, through a convex lens, as without, certainly indicates hypermetropia.

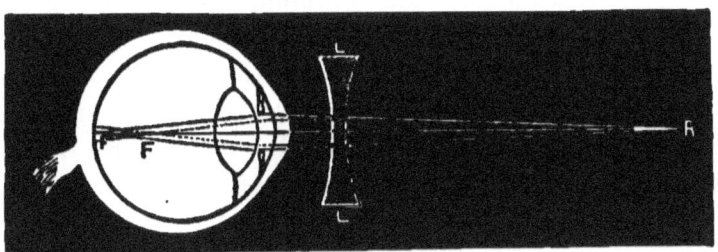

FIG. 23.—Section of myopic eye.
R, the origin of divergent rays of light ; F, the focus of these in front of retina ; LL, concave lens to be worn by myope ; F', focus of rays of light on retina, showing influence of L.

Myopia is essentially due to the soft and yielding character of the tunic of some children's eyes, enabling the pressure of the muscles during accommodation to elongate the globe. The condition when started may remain stationary, but in some cases the continuance of the cause increases the elongation of the globe. This may be followed by stretching and atrophy of the choroid, or even detachment of the retina, and other evil consequences, resulting in partial or complete destruction of vision.

The tendency to short-sight is generally strongly hereditary, but it may be acquired, and it is chiefly during school-life that this occurs. Jäger, in 1861, first called attention to the remarkable development of myopia during school-life. Dr. Cohn, of Breslau, in 1865, took up the subject. Having examined the eyes of 10,060 children, he found 1,072 myopic, 239 hypermetropic, 23 astigmatic, and 396 whose vision was impaired from the effects of previous disease. As his testing was by lenses only, he probably underrated the myopia. In elementary village-schools he found 1·4 per cent. of myopia, in town elementary-schools, 6·7 per cent. ; in intermediate schools, 10·3 per cent. ; high schools, 19·7 ; and in gymnasia, 26·2 per cent. Among medical students he found the proportion in the first year of study 52 per cent., in the last year 64 per cent. At Tübingen, Gärtner found that of 600 theological students, 79 per cent. were myopic.

Although Germany has until lately had the greatest prevalence of defects of vision, it has by no means a monopoly of them. In all the cases investigated, the fact comes out that the youngest classes have the fewest myopics, and the oldest most. Drs. E. G. Loring and R. H. Derby, of New York, found that in the lowest classes 3·5 and in the highest 26·78 per cent were myopic.

The statistics furnished by the Philadelphia Committee, of which Dr. Risley was chairman, are peculiarly valuable, as a complete examination of the eye (barring the use of Atropine) was made in each case. 2,422 eyes were examined by the committee, and 174 afterwards by Dr. Jackson, of West Chester, on the same plan, each case requiring on an average, twenty-eight minutes' examination.

The accompanying chart, from Mr. B. Carter's pamphlet on "Eyesight in Schools," shows the result. (Fig. 24). The horizontal lines give the percentages, the vertical lines the different classes. The myopia was found to increase from 4·27 per cent. in primary classes (average age, 8½ years) to 19·33 per cent. in normal classes, while the hypermetropia diminished from 88·11 per cent. to 66·84 per cent., the proportion of normal vision (emmetropia) remaining nearly stationary. It is evident, from the statistics just advanced, that school-life has, under conditions which commonly prevail, a most deleterious influence on eyesight.

Astigmatism is a condition of the eyes in which the curvature of the cornea is not uniform, and consequently rays of light passing through it in different meridians have a different focus. The lines running in a given direction look blurred—as all the horizontal or all the upright, &c. Children suffering from this condition often appear stupid or inattentive, because there is in this defect what has been aptly called "slow sight"; a word is not recognised quickly on

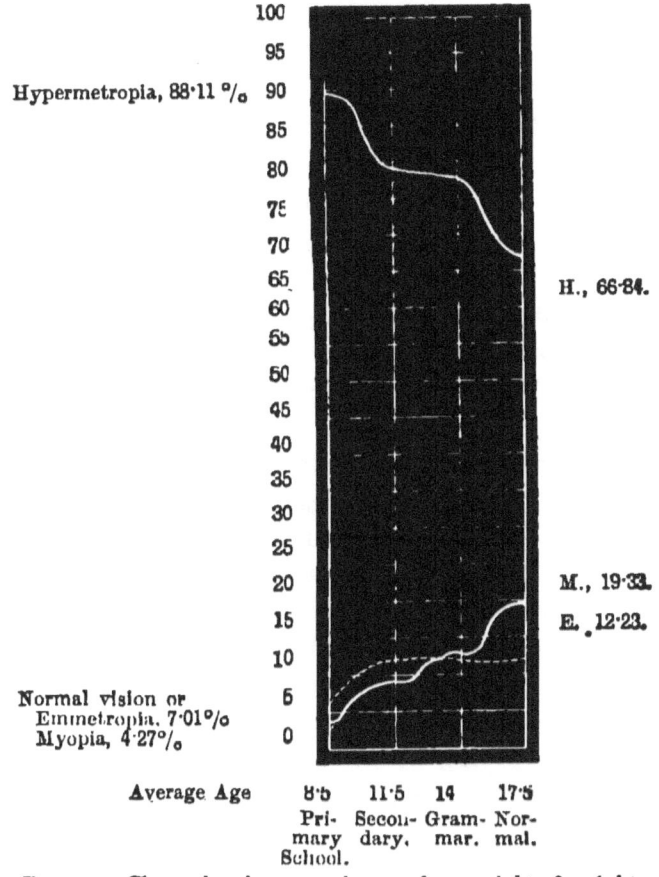

FIG. 24.—Chart showing prevalence of near-sight, far-sight, and normal vision at different ages.

first sight, but "it seems to come to them afterwards." The defect is commonly ascribed to near-sightedness, but ordinary convex lenses will not remedy it; lenses, the curve of which is specially adapted to each meridian of the eye, being required.

The causes at work during school-life which tend to produce defects of vision may be classed under the five following heads:

(1.) The *prolonged exertion* of the eyes involved in seeing *near objects*. School-work usually lasts from four to six hours, and the home-lessons sometimes nearly as long. During a great part of this time, the accommodating apparatus of the child's eyes is being strained; the tissues of the eyes being soft and compressible, evil results are apt to occur, especially when there is a hereditary tendency to defects of vision. Three hours' good work is always better than five hours of indifferent work.

The posture of the scholar is very important. He should not be allowed to lean forward with a bent head. In writing we have a good instance of the principles involved, and the practice to be followed. The movements required are of a complicated character, and, like the complicated movements concerned in speech and walking, should be automatically performed. In fact, the more automatic and the less conscious the movements become, the greater is the degree of precision attained. Hence, as in piano-playing, where the pupil is required to look at the music and not at the keys, the pupil who is writing should be required to sit erect, and directly facing the desk, and should fix his attention on the matter to be written, rather than on the movements of the fingers. The desk should be at a proper angle to the eyes, and the eyes should not be allowed to come nearer than 12 inches from the book or slate. The copy-book should be aslant, to allow for the bend in the writing; otherwise a twisted position is necessary.

(2) An *inadequate amount of light*, or an ill-directed light, causes an undue strain on the eyes. The amount of window area required, and the direction of the light admitted, have been already discussed (page 18). It is probable that the preparation of home-lessons in semi-darkness is responsible for much injury to the eyes.

Cohn in his investigations found that the narrower the street in which the school stood, the higher the opposite houses, and the lower the storey in which lessons were given, the greater the number of cases of myopia among elementary scholars. He proposed that 30 square inches of glass (not including the window frames) should be allowed for every square foot of floor-area.

(3.) *Badly printed text and other books* produce the same result. The *type* should be clear and large, Roman being much better than Gothic type. The construction of such letters as *h* and *b*, *v* and *n* should be especially precise.

The following words represent well-known sizes of type :—
Double Pica.   *Great Primer.*   *Pica.*
No type smaller than Pica should
Small Pica. Bourgeois. Minion. Pearl. Brilliant.
be used while teaching children to read.

Cohn proposes that the type of ordinary journals should be 4 mm. or ⅙ inch in height, though M. Javal thinks it may be allowed to be 2 mm. The thickness of down and up-strokes, the spaces between letters and words and between lines, and the length of lines all require attention.

Letter-press derived from a *worn-out fount* gives an imperfect impression of the letters. The loops of *a* and *e*, of *b d p g* are apt to form a black spot ; long letters become broken, and fine up-strokes are imperceptible.

Books for children should not be too large and heavy, the spaces between the letters and between words and lines should be relatively wide, and the lines not too long. The reading or writing-book should be placed at a distance of twelve to fifteen inches from the eyes. The most agreeable tint of paper is a cream-colour or a pale blue. It is inadvisable to gloss the sheets, as this produces a dazzling reflection.

I

It is important that too small a handwriting should not be allowed, and that neither writing nor reading should be permitted in the dim light of evening.

Pale ink and greasy slates are very trying to the eyes.

The letters on many maps in schools are most trying to the eyes, the lettering not only being fine, but the maps having often been printed from old and worn plates. Maps should contain as few data as possible, teaching by wall-maps and outline maps being preferable. In writing lessons, the character of the writing material used is of some importance, especially on dull winter days. Thus the furthest distance at which a specimen of slate-pencil writing was recognisable, as compared with a specimen of lead-pencil writing of the same size, was as 7 to 8, while the ratio of lead-pencil to pen and ink legibility was 7 to 8, and of slate writing to pen and ink 3 to 4. The bearing of this on the hygiene of the eye is evident; pen and ink writing should be used where possible. Also pale ink, or ink which turns black only after a time, should be abolished from school.

(4.) *Needlework* is a too frequent cause of defective vision in girls. Sewing is more trying to the eyes than any work that boys have to do. In ordinary coarse calico there are about 70 threads to an inch, and what is considered good work consists in taking up 4 threads, 2 in front and 2 behind the cotton; while in moderately fine linen, as a shirt-front, there are 120 threads to an inch, so that the sempstress has to work to $\frac{1}{60}$ inch, a much smaller distance than the finest print.

The sewing required of children should be neat and accurate, but not too fine, and sewing should not be prolonged, nor undertaken in a bad light. Where possible, the light should come from above for needlework, as for drawing lessons, and such lessons should be avoided by gas-light. Needlework and drawing and writing lessons should always, preferably, be given during the brightest hours of the day. Lace-work taxes the eyes severely, and may lead to absolute loss of vision. Working at night on black dresses is most injurious. Scarlet materials are somewhat trying to the eyes, and are not allowed under the London School Board ; blue is to be preferred.

(5.) The condition of *the general health* produced by insufficient exercise or food, and the influence of a vitiated atmosphere, powerfully favour the production of defective vision. So, likewise, does the occurrence of catarrhal or other affections of the eye, as after measles, diphtheria, and scarlet fever.

CHAPTER XVIII.

COMMUNICABLE DISEASES IN SCHOOLS.

Moral Duty of Parents and Medical Men.—Symptoms of Onset of Infectious Diseases.—Rules for Guidance of Teachers.—Duration of Infection.—Isolation of Healthy Members of Household.—Diseases from Insanitary Schools.—Question of Closing Schools for Epidemics.—Management of Infectious Diseases in Boarding Schools.—Other Communicable Diseases.—Ringworm.—Itch.

THE question of infection is not of such vital moment in a day-school as in a boarding-school, but still it is of the utmost importance that both teachers and parents should be cognisant of the general facts bearing on this question. An error on the part of the parent, in sending a child to school too early during convalescence, or on the part of the teacher, in failing to recognise the early symptoms of a fever, may lead to rapid spread of the disease, and a thorough disorganisation of school-life.

On the part of the parent or guardian an increased sense of moral obligation is much needed. .Too often the mother is only anxious that the child should return to school as speedily as possible, regardless of the evil consequences to his schoolfellows; or again, the existence of a case of infectious disease in the house is concealed, in order that other children from the same house may not be forbidden to attend school.

On the other hand, the teacher must never relax rules for particular cases. A fixed time must elapse before return is allowed (see below), and this must be adhered to even though, in exceptional cases, an earlier return would be unattended with danger.

Family doctors should, in like manner, have regard to the important and wide-spread interests involved, and always name, as the earliest period for return to school, a date when every possibility of infection is past.

We have briefly to consider in this chapter—

(*a*) Infectious diseases communicable from one child to another.

(*b*) Diseases, like typhoid fever, which are due to local insanitary conditions, and

(*c*) Certain contagious diseases of the skin and eye.

Specific infectious diseases may arise in connection with school-life, from the attendance of children at school who are either (1) suffering from the early symptoms of, or (2) are convalescing from infectious disease, or (3) who although healthy come from homes in which infectious disease is present.

The first and second of these causes, unfortunately, not infrequently exist, especially in the case of measles, whooping cough, mumps, scarlet fever, and diphtheria. It is essential to the elimination of these causes, that teachers and parents should be familiar with (1) the symptoms indicating the onset, and (2) the duration of infection in these diseases.

Onset of Infectious Diseases.—In each infectious disease an interval elapses between the reception of the specific poison, and the development of the earliest symptoms, known as the *period of incubation*, or hatching. During this time the patient may be in fair health and is *not infectious*, according to the majority of medical authorities.

With the onset of the earliest symptoms, he becomes a centre of infection, though usually not so dangerously as a few days later. The period of incubation of the various fevers is shown in the following table:—

Disease.	Begins usually on the	But may possibly be at any period between
Scarlet Fever.........	4th day.	1 & 7 days.
Diphtheria.............	2nd „	2 & 5 „
Small pox............	12th „	1 & 14 „
Chicken pox	14th „	10 & 18 „
Typhus Fever	12th „	1 & 21 „
Typhoid Fever.	21st „	1 & 28 „
Measles	12th-14th „	10 & 14 „
Rötheln	14th „	12 & 18 „
Mumps................	19th „	16 & 24 „
Whooping Cough...	14th „	7 & 14 „

Following the period of incubation, come the premonitory symptoms, which usually are somewhat sudden in onset.

In *Scarlet Fever* the child, as a rule, vomits and becomes extremely feverish, at the same time complaining of sore throat. Any child at school who is sick, and has a hot dry skin, should be immediately sent home. Within 24 hours a punctiform red rash appears on the chest, soon becoming a scarlet blush, and spreading to other parts. Some cases are so slight that they may come to school throughout, and be discovered only by the occurrence of peeling or dropsy due to chill affecting the kidneys, which may occur after the mildest cases.

In *Diphtheria*, after a day or two of languor and sore throat, white patches appear on the tonsils and contiguous parts, which in severe cases join together to form a continuous membrane. Smaller white patches, due to the condition called ulcerated throat (follicular tonsillitis), are often confused with the much more severe disease, diphtheria. Both, however, are extremely contagious by inhalation of the breath, and, undoubtedly, are frequently spread in schools, when mild cases have been overlooked. The presence of sore throat and feverishness, would always justify the teacher in sending a scholar home, with a note to its parent.

Small-pox comes on with severe pain in the loins, sickness, and shivering. At the end of 48 hours, a hard, pimply rash appears, and then the patient usually feels better for a while. A patient with ordinary small-pox, would be too ill to attend school ; but the modified small-pox, which occurs in those partially protected by vaccination, is a much milder complaint, and in one case, known to the writer, a boy attended school with it, being supposed to have a " spring rash." In such a case small-pox would be likely to spread among those who had been imperfectly or unsuccessfully vaccinated.

Chicken-pox may come on with hardly any premonitory symptoms, except slight feverishness. The rash comes out in 24 hours—at first pimples, but speedily becoming clear vesicles. There may be some difficulty in diagnosing from modified small-pox, though the rash in the latter seldom or never appears on the scalp, as it does in chicken-pox.

Measles comes on with all the symptoms of a severe cold in the head, with an unusual amount of fever. At the end of 72 hours, red blotchy spots appear on the face, hands, and other parts, and rapidly spread, tending to assume crescentic arrangements.

Rötheln or *German Measles* has a rash somewhat like that of measles. There is no nasal catarrh, however, and always a sore throat, similar to, but less severe than, that of scarlet-fever. It is always a slight complaint, and is sometimes mistaken for the *rose-rash* due to indigestion, &c., a mistake which may lead to serious results in large schools. In all doubtful cases, the safest plan is to act as if it were the infectious complaint.

Mumps comes on with feverishness and pain near the ear, followed by enlargement of the parotid salivary gland. This causes bulging out at the side of the neck and in *front of the ear*, by which means it can be distinguished from glandular enlargement due to other causes.

As a rule both sides are affected, but occasionally only one.

Whooping Cough is a disease in which the characteristic cough does not come on for a week or two, but the cough appears to be simply due to bronchial catarrh. It is unfortunate that during this unrecognisable stage (unless by the history of infection) the disease can be communicated to others. At the end of 7 to 14 days the patient begins to cough till he is out of breath, and then draws in his breath with a peculiar crowing noise or whoop. Every teacher should be familiar with this whoop, and send any child home who has it, or who even without it has *a cough severe enough to make him sick.*

What has been said about the onset of common infectious diseases may be summarised for the practical use of the teacher as follows :—

(1.) Whenever a child appears at school with a suspicious-looking rash, or if he is sick or becomes feverish and ill, send him home at once with a note to his parents.

(2.) A bad sore-throat, with feverishness, might indicate scarlet fever, diphtheria, German measles, or a simple sore-throat. In any case send the patient home, and ask the mother to keep him away from school until the true nature of the complaint becomes certain.

(3.) If a child is suffering from a severe cold, with sneezing and redness of the eyes, it may mean an influenza co'd or measles. As both are contagious, the child should be sent home.

(4.) A swelling in front of, and below, the ear, nearly always means mumps; while a paroxysmal cough, making the child sick or bleed at the nose, or become blue in the face, generally means whooping-cough. In all doubtful cases, *act as though it were certain* that the case was an infectious one.

Duration of Infection.—It is important to know at what period, after the onset of an infectious disease, a child may return to school. This should theoretically coincide with the end of the period of infection, but as it is wise in all cases to allow a margin, we have given the duration of infection, and the period at which return to school may be allowed, in separate columns in the following table. In the fourth column is given the period which must elapse before a child, who has been exposed to infection, may, in the absence of symptoms, be allowed to return to school, assuming that in the interval he has been completely isola ed from any source of infection. This, again, should theoretically coincide with the longest corresponding period of incubation given in the last table (page 118), but it is well to allow a margin for the symptoms, if coming on, to become fully developed.

It must be clearly borne in mind that the date of cessation of the *patient's* infection is stated in the following table. It is assumed that all wearing-apparel has been disinfected, and likewise the room occupied by the child. Sometimes a child is taken ill in a particular dress, and resumes this on returning to school, thus carrying the infection with him.

A scholar who has been suffering from infectious disease should never be re-admitted to school without a medical certificate of freedom from infection. If this certificate assumes freedom from infection at an earlier period than the one

SCHOOL HYGIENE.

Disease.	Duration of Infection.	Date at which School attendance may be resumed.	Duration of Quarantine of children exposed to Infection.
Scarlet Fever	From 5 to 8 weeks; ceases when all peeling of the skin has been completed.	Not less than 6 weeks from the beginning of the rash and then only if no peeling or sore-throat is present.	14 days.
Diphtheria	From 14 to 21 days.	Not less than 3 weeks, & not then if strength not recovered, or if any sore throat or any discharge from nose, eyes, ears, &c.	12 days.
Small pox and Chicken pox	About 4 to 5 weeks.	When every scab has fallen off.	18 days.
Measles	From 2 to 4 weeks, when all cough and branny shedding of skin has ceased.	When all desquamation is completed, not less than 3 weeks from beginning of rash.	16 days.
Rötheln	10 to 14 days.	From 2 to 3 weeks varying with the attack.	16 days.
Mumps	14 to 21 days, from the beginning	Four weeks from the beginning, if all swelling has disappeared.	24 days.
Whooping Cough	6 weeks from the beginning of whooping, or when the cough has quite ceased.	In about 8 weeks.	21 days.
Typhus & Typhoid Fevers	4 to 5 weeks.	When strength sufficient.	28 days.

named in the preceding table, the question should be referred to another doctor, preferably one to be attached as an official adviser to the school. It sometimes happens, for instance, that children are sent back to school with a medical certificate of freedom from infection at the end of fourteen days from the beginning of mumps, which is at least a week too early.

The admission to school of apparently healthy children from infected households should always be forbidden, because of the possibility of their carrying the infection in their clothes, or of their coming to school while having the disease in a latent form or an unrecognised stage. As soon as the teacher knows of the existence of a case of infectious disease, he should at once exclude from school every child living in the same house. The Sanitary Authorities as a rule communicate with the teacher, instructing him not to admit to school any children from an infected house. Except in towns where the compulsory notification of infectious diseases is enforced, the proportion of cases known to Sanitary Officials is, however, very small, and the teacher is consequently warned from this source only in a minority of cases. The London School Board has issued instructions to its teachers, that they shall inform the Local Sanitary Authority of all cases coming to their knowledge. This regulation seems to be seldom obeyed. The enforcement of the compulsory notification of infectious diseases by parents, would enable teachers and health-officers to work more efficiently together, to their mutual advantage.

All the children in an infected house should be kept away from school while the infectious disease continues, and for a given period of quarantine afterwards which is stated in the last table. The quarantine-period must be assumed to start from the end of the longest possible period of infection of the last person who has been ill in the house. Thus, referring to the table, it will be seen that, after scarlet fever, an exposed child must not return to school for 8 *plus* 2 weeks; after diphtheria, 21 *plus* 12 days; after mumps, 21 *plus* 24 days, &c.

This may seem an unnecessarily long period, but the only way to avoid possible infection, is to adhere rigidly to it where children have remained *in the same house* as their sick brothers. Of course, if the healthy children have been removed to another house, and no possible communication is allowed, then only the period of quarantine given in the last column of the table on page 122 need be insisted on.

In some cases, disease has been acquired from some local *unsanitary condition of the school-premises*. Bad drains or closets may give rise to typhoid fever or diphtheria, as may likewise a tainted water-supply. In the former case, the school should be closed during the necessary repairs; in the latter, the water-supply should be cut off. Bad ventilation may serve to intensify an imported infection, and increase its virulence; and so may, likewise, a dirty condition of the walls and floors of the school.

When any child attending school has been discovered to be suffering from an infectious disease, he should be sent home, the other children sent into the playground, and then the windows widely opened and the floor freely sprinkled with some disinfecting solution, as carbolic acid, 1 to 60 of water.

The necessity of closing schools for infectious disease but rarely arises. Where prompt information is received by the local sanitary authority of the occurrence of infectious cases, it is rarely, if ever, necessary to close a school, as the children of infected households can be kept away.

In certain exceptional cases it may be advisable to close a school. Thus: (1) If the attendance at the school is greatly reduced by a severe epidemic (of measles, for instance). preventing the continuance of a regular course of study. (2) In sparsely-populated rural districts, where children rarely meet except at school, closing the school may effectually check the spread of an epidemic, though it is of little use in towns or large villages, where children play together out of school-hours. (3) School should be closed for a few days or weeks to remedy local sanitary defects. If a drain is opened during school-hours, children crowd about to see what is done, and may thus receive the germs of diphtheria or typhoid fever.

To prevent the origin and spread of infectious diseases in large public and boarding schools, some further precautions are required. The sanitary conditions of the school should be perfect, the water and milk supplies above suspicion, and the school should, if possible, have its own laundry.

The school infirmary or sanatorium should preferably be entirely separate from the rest of the school, and should have rooms for distinct cases of fever, and other rooms in which doubtful cases may be watched until their true character

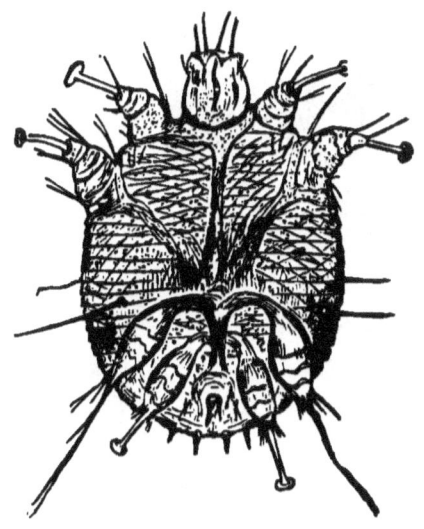

FIG. 25.—The itch insect. (After Startin.)

becomes evident.   The importance of not leaving any case of illness accompanied by a rise of temperature in the common dormitories cannot be exaggerated.   It is generally by means of doubtful or ill-marked cases of fever that infection is spread; and in some cases it is necessary to wait and see whether peeling occurs before a correct diagnosis can be made.

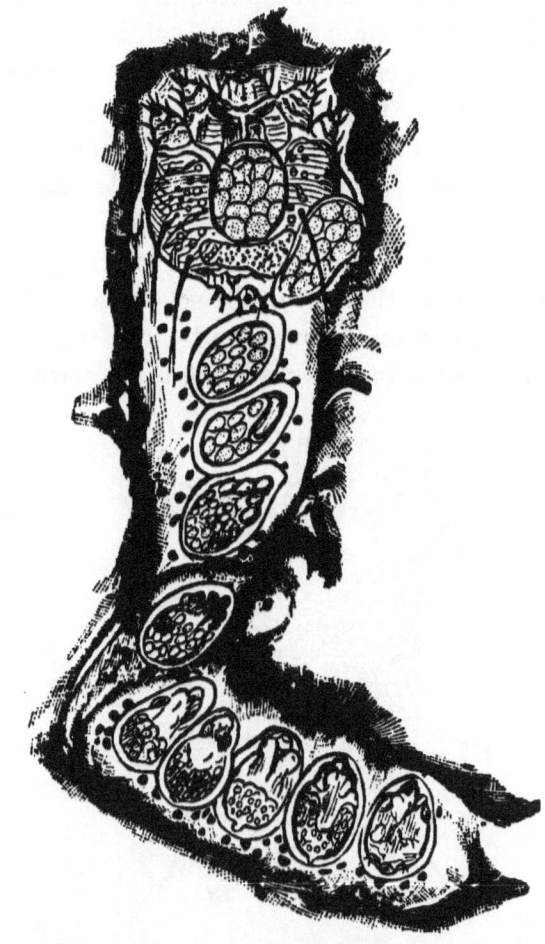

FIG. 26.—A burrow formed by the itch-insect in the epidermis, showing the mature animal and nine eggs in course of development. Highly magnified. (After Startin.)

The sanatorium should have nurses' rooms, a small kitchen, bath, and water-closets complete in itself, and isolated from the rest of the school. When a separate building is impossible, the top floor of the house should be occupied, and in this case even more stringent regulations are required. One medical attendant should attend all the cases of sickness in a school. Where the medical responsibility is divided, infection is much more apt to spread.

Certificates should be demanded from the guardians or parents of children on their return after vacations, stating that there has been no known exposure to infection for at least three weeks. Where no such statement can be obtained, the pupil should be placed in quarantine; he should have a warm bath, strong carbolic soap being used, and his clothes and books should be baked. In large schools it may be advisable to have a disinfecting oven, Washington Lyon's, in which superheated steam is employed, being the best for this purpose.

Other Communicable Diseases.—*Scabies* or *Itch* shows itself in the form of an irritable rash, most frequently seen between the roots of the fingers and in the bends of joints, especially at the wrist. It is due to the rapid multiplication of a minute insect not unlike a cheese-mite (Fig. 25), the female of which forms oblique burrows in the epidermis, laying eggs which hatch in about 14 days (Fig. 26). The rash simulates eczema, and is liable to spread all over the body if its true nature is not detected. It is very contagious, and no child who has had it should be allowed to return to school without a medical certificate, and until his clothes have been baked or washed in boiling water.

Ringworm is due to the growth on the skin of a microscopic fungus (Fig. 27). Minute spores become detached from the growth, and thus infection is carried elsewhere to the same person or to others by means of change of hats or bonnets, or by towels or brushes, or actual contact. Hairdressers occasionally communicate ringworm, and so do hatters by trying on numerous caps. It is as morally wrong to send a child with ringworm to a hairdresser or hatter as if he were suffering from scarlet fever. The frequency of ringworm is shown by the experience of Christ's Hospital, London, in which children from all parts of the country, and all grades of middle-class society are

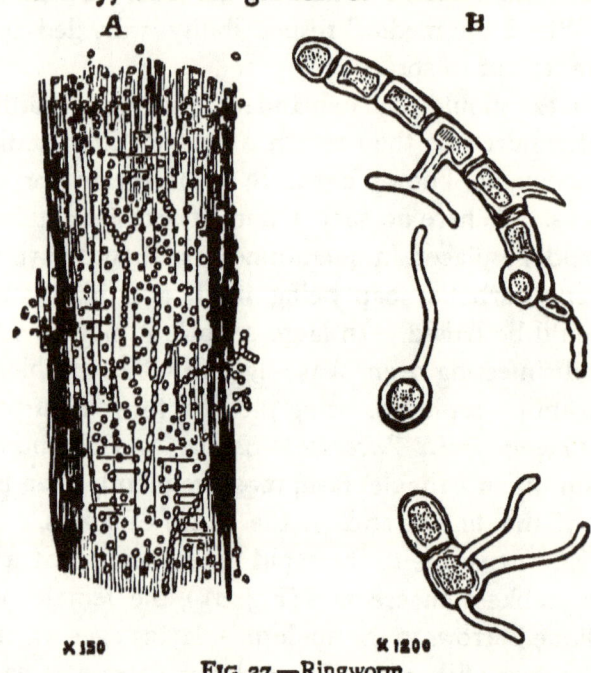

FIG. 27.—Ringworm.

A, a hair, showing filtration with the growth, magnified 150 times.
B, a portion of the fungus magnified 1,200 times. (Bristowe's Medicine.)

admitted. In the ten years, 1875-84, 1812 children, aged from 8 to 10 years, all supposed to be free from ringworm, were examined for the first time, and 145 cases were detected, or about 8 per cent. of all children admitted.

On the bare skin, ring-like patches with raised margins are formed, the ring gradually widening out if not interfered with. On the scalp similar patches are formed, but the fungus extends down to the roots of the hairs, and obstinately remains there, even when the superficial parts have been apparently cured. It frequently happens that such children are allowed to return to school, the disease breaking out again, and causing infection of other children. It is quite a mistake to suppose that ringworm is necessarily cured when the hair begins to grow on the diseased places. A case can be regarded as cured only when a medical man, after having carefully examined the whole scalp in a good light and scrutinised every suspicious spot with a lens, has found no broken-off stumpy hairs (often not protruding more than $\frac{1}{16}$ to $\frac{1}{8}$ inch).

It is unfortunately a fact that many children recovering from ringworm are certified by indiscreet medical men to be free from infection, when a more careful examination discovers numerous hairs in which the fungus is still alive. One commonly hears the remark that "the ringworm is better, but has left a scurfy condition of the head behind." The teacher may take it as a practical rule in such cases which will very seldom be found to err, that the *scurfy condition* indicates a phase of ringworm which *is still infectious*. The power of infection may continue even when one or two years of this scurfy condition have elapsed.

Catarrhal Ophthalmia is marked by redness of the eyes and free muco-purulent discharge. It lasts about 14 days, and is chiefly important because it is contagious.

Chronic Granular Ophthalmia is also contagious, and all cases should be isolated, and the use of the same towels, or water, forbidden. Badly-ventilated dormitories, insufficient food, and general unhygienic conditions with the promiscuous use of towels, are chiefly instrumental in producing it. Those of an Irish nationality seem to be particularly prone to suffer from it.

Scald Head (Contagious Impetigo) is common in underfed children. It may spread to other children, under similar conditions; and such children should therefore be excluded from school.

In concluding this long but important chapter, brief allusion should be made to Chorea, and Hysteria, which are communicable by imitation and sympathy, and for this reason should be excluded from school. Every teacher should be able to recognise the jerky twitchings, the shuffling of feet, the contortions of face and twitching of eyelids, which characterise Chorea (St. Vitus's Dance) and children suffering from this, require prolonged rest from school-work.

Hysteria is chiefly of importance in girls' schools. It assumes various forms, and may occasionally simulate either a simple faint or an epileptic fit. It is distinguished from the former by the absence of the extreme pallor of face and lips, which characterises fainting; and from the latter by the fact that the hysterical patient is usually not completely unconscious, as shown by the attempts to attract sympathy and attention, and by the flinching which occurs when the white of the eye is touched with the point of a finger. The patient should be treated firmly, though kindly, and not allowed to attract too much attention.

CHAPTER XIX.

SCHOOL ACCIDENTS.

Importance of "First Aid."—Fainting.—Fits.—Suffocation.—Drowning.—Foreign Bodies.—Stings and Bites.—Wounds.—Hæmorrhage.—Burns.—Fractures, Dislocations, Sprains, and Contusions.—Football.

THE extreme utility of "First Aid" to the injured, is shown by the popularity which the St. John Ambulance lectures have attained. To teachers, the knowledge of "First Aid" is particularly useful, for, in addition to the numerous accidents that occur in connection with school games, instances of children having fits or faints, or hæmorrhage, are by no means uncommon. Panic, which is the result of ignorance, and, still more important, injury to health and limb, might frequently be prevented by the application of the simple rules of treatment which will be laid down in this chapter.

It must not be supposed that we are encouraging teachers to take upon themselves the sole treatment of serious cases, although we may have to describe the treatment of such cases in detail. But valuable time is frequently lost before a medical man arrives, and it is therefore highly important that the teacher should know what to do in the interval. Hence a not unsuitable heading for this chapter would be—"Until the doctor comes."

Fainting in schools which are ill-ventilated and over-heated, is not infrequent. The patient should be laid on his back, with his head low; all tight clothing should be removed from his neck; crowding round him should be avoided, and, if possible, he should be placed in a free current of air, near an open door. Do not attempt to pour anything down the throat while the patient remains unconscious, otherwise choking may result.

Fits may occur in school. In boys' schools, epileptic fits occur; in girls' schools, hysterical fits may likewise occur.

In epilepsy, during the convulsions, the patient should be laid gently on the floor, and prevented from biting his tongue, if possible. All tight clothing should be removed, and no further attempt at active treatment made.

In hysteria, as a rule, the patient is not quite unconscious; she sobs considerably, and is evidently in a highly emotional condition. She will not allow the ball of her eye to be touched with the finger without flinching, unlike an epileptic patient. Hysterical patients should be removed from the school as soon as possible, as a bad example of this kind is likely to spread. Their morbid condition should not be fed by over-attention or indulgence.

Suffocation is occasionally imminent from a marble or cherry stone, or similar substance, being held in the mouth, and then suddenly sucked down into the larynx. Such an accident is always serious, and a doctor should be immediately called, the messenger being instructed to tell him the nature of the accident in order that no time may be lost. In the meantime, the only safe measure is to put the finger to the back of the throat, in the hope that the foreign body may be reached. Even if it is not reached, vomiting is commonly excited, and this may dislodge it. The child should not be inverted until the doctor arrives, as, if it is not successful, the symptoms may be aggravated.

SCHOOL ACCIDENTS. 133

Apparent Drowning is a not infrequent accident, especially in country districts during half-holidays, and the teacher should instruct his scholars as to the plan to be followed in such an emergency.

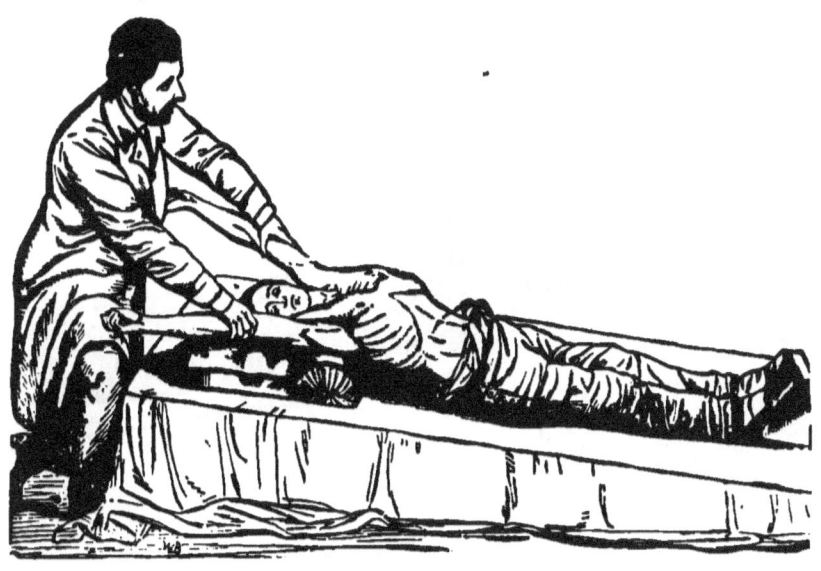

FIG. 28 —The inspiratory movement in artificial respiration.

The apparently-drowned boy should be placed on the bank, his mouth cleansed from mud, &c., and his tongue drawn forward out of the mouth.* A folded coat should be placed under his head and shoulders, so as to give firm support. Next, the boy's arms should be grasped near the elbows by the operator, who stands over the boy, facing towards his feet. The arms should be drawn over the boy's head, and then pressed down firmly against the sides of his chest. (Figs. 28 and 29.) This manipulation should be repeated regularly about fifteen times a minute, taking care not to perform the movements hurriedly. The upward movement expands the chest, while the pressure of the arms on the chest causes expulsion of air from it. In this

* See Note I., page 140.

way inspiration and expiration are imitated, and the natural process of respiration may in favourable cases be restored.

At the same time, other persons should secure warm and dry

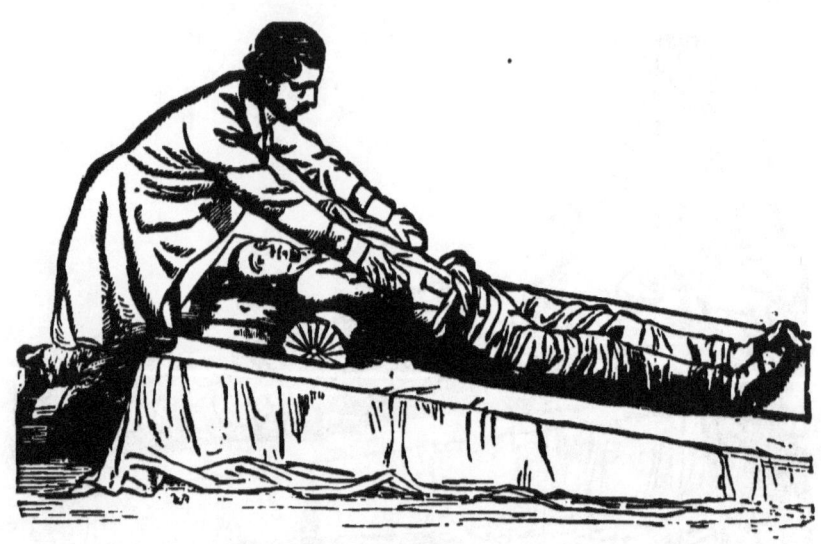

FIG. 29.—The expiratory movement in artificial respiration.

blankets and hot bottles, and should rub the legs steadily, so as to help the circulation and keep up the temperature of the body. The artificial respiration is, however, the most important point, and should not be intermitted until natural attempts at breathing occur, or until half-an-hour has elapsed without sign of recovery.

Foreign Bodies are occasionally pushed by mischievous children into the ear or nostril. In the latter case they can usually be seen and seized by a pair of tweezers, or hooked down by a fine wire hoop.* In the former case simple syringing with warm water will frequently wash out the foreign matter. If it is a pea, however, syringing is better omitted, as the pea may swell and thus become more firmly impacted.

Minute particles of dust, &c., frequently set up great irrita-

* See Note II., page 140.

tion in the eye. Try to invert the upper eyelid, and then the speck can usually be seen, and removed with the corner of a pocket-handkerchief. If it cannot be seen, drop a little castor-oil into the eye, keep the eye closed and immobile by means of a wet compress over it, and, if relief is not obtained in a few hours, seek further advice.

If a needle becomes imbedded under the skin, the affected part should be kept fixed, and a surgeon seen. Thorns and splinters may usually be removed by cutting through the top skin (epidermis) with a sharp and clean knife, and then seizing the fragment with a pair of tweezers. If the splinter is under the finger-nail, its removal is much more difficult, and the teacher will seldom have skill or courage to cut down the nail as is sometimes necessary.

The *Stings* of bees and wasps are best relieved by first bathing with hot water and squeezing out the poison, and then applying a strong solution of common cooking soda to the affected parts. The same treatment holds good for nettle-stings.

The *Bite* of a dog is not in itself serious, unless the dog is mad.* As, however, the fact cannot at once be ascertained, it is wise to adopt the necessary precautions in every case. The wound should be bathed with hot water and thoroughly sponged. It is also desirable to increase bleeding from the wound by enlarging it with a sharp pocket-knife. Lunar caustic is of little service, but as most schools have some strong nitric acid on the premises, this should be carefully applied to the wound by means of a penholder dipped in the acid, any excess of the acid having been first removed from the penholder.

Wounds of varying degree and severity are very apt to occur in connection with school-life. The wounded part should be laid bare, and the wound thoroughly washed with cold water, in order to remove any grit or other foreign

---

* To make sure of this point, it is wiser not to shoot the dog until the doubt is fully solved.

matter that may have entered it. Then the edges should be brought as near together as possible, and a pad of linen moistened with cold water should be applied by means of a bandage. The patient should be placed in such a position that the edges of the wound will not be strained; thus, if the wound is on the cheek, speaking and chewing should be avoided; if on the leg, walking must not be allowed. Punctured wounds, from knives, &c., may be more serious and in all doubtful cases a medical man should be seen.

Abrasions, in which the skin is rubbed off, are best treated by washing carefully with cold water, and then applying some Friar's balsam or collodion. For wounds and abrasions, sticking-plaster should never be applied alone. It nearly always sets up irritation and causes the wound to suppurate.

Swollen glands are apt to occur after a wound or whitlow, or other injury. Thus, a swelling under the armpit may occur from a poisoned finger. Such a condition requires careful attention, rather to the cause of the enlarged glands, than to the glands themselves. Enlarged glands in the neck are not infrequently due to lice in the head or a discharge from the ears, or sore eyes, or a rash on the head or face. Given that these conditions are removed, the enlarged glands disappear, unless some disorder of the general health co-exists.

Hæmorrhage is due to the rupture of a blood-vessel. This may be due to a wound, or may come from the lungs, nose, or other parts, independently of external injury.

Arterial bleeding is the most serious, and is distinguished from venous or capillary bleeding, by its greater amount, by the bright scarlet colour of the blood, and by the fact that it comes out in intermittent jets, corresponding to the beats of the heart.

Venous or capillary bleeding can always be controlled by placing a linen pad on the wound, and firmly bandaging it in its place.

To control arterial bleeding, the same measure is usually successful, only the pad must be made firm and hard, and tightly bound in its place. If a main artery is divided, as shown by the great spurting of blood, a firm pad may be held firmly pressed by the two thumbs over the wound until further aid can be obtained. If the teacher knows the course of the main blood-vessels in the limb, he may stop the hæmorrhage by pressing his thumb over the main artery higher up the limb; but as a rule, he will probably be more successful by trusting to a firm pad kept forcibly pressed over the wound itself.

An elevated position of the limb will help to stop bleeding from it, and a flexed position of the joint next above the wounded part has a similar effect. Thus, with a severe wound in the palm of the hand, apply a pad firmly over the wound, bend the elbow, and keep the whole arm raised. If coughing or vomiting of blood occurs, keep the patient perfectly quiet, and give nothing except ice to suck, and obtain medical aid at once. In bleeding from the nose, apply iced compresses to the nape of the neck, and syringe the nose out with iced water. If this does not answer, put some alum or tannin in the water to be injected into the nostril, or pack the nostril with a large wad of cotton soaked in alum-water. If the bleeding still continues, a powder containing 30 grains of bromide of potassium may be given in water, and repeated in half an hour if necessary. This seldom fails to stop the hæmorrhage.

Burns are apt to occur in connection with open fires or hot water pipes. The best immediate application is probably a linen cloth soaked in a saturated solution of common cooking soda, which very quickly relieves the pain and burning.

The following injuries are most apt to occur in connection with football, though occasionally from cricket or in the gymnasium:

Fractures are recognised by inability to use the affected limb, shortening and alteration in its shape, and a grating sound when an attempt is made to move it. There is no urgency about treating a broken limb before the arrival of a surgeon. If it is necessary, however, to remove him indoors, the limb should first be secured in splints, and he should be carried on an improvised stretcher. Splints may be improvised by taking long pieces of a box-lid, or an umbrella; or for children, brown paper folded up so as to be stiff and rigid.

Dislocations are liable to be confused with fractures, but the limb is more fixed than in fracture, and there is no grating sound or movement. The fact that the injury is obviously near a joint helps to a diagnosis, though sometimes fractures may occur close to a joint. Any attempt at replacing the dislocated bone by an unskilled person is dangerous.

Sprains are best treated by bandaging immediately, and applying spirit and water, or some quite warm, soothing lotion. The part should be kept immobile, and the after-treatment requires great care.

Contusions, as from a kick on the shin or a blow in the eye, result in the effusion of blood under the skin (as in the "black eye"). The effusion may be minimised, and its absorption helped by a cold evaporating lotion.

More serious accidents occasionally happen in cricket and football. In cricket, a fatal result has occasionally followed a blow behind the ear by the cricket-ball. It is difficult to suggest precautions that would prevent the possibility of this accident.

In football, a blow or kick over the abdomen or chest may cause sudden death, or, short of this, complete collapse, which in some cases requires several weeks before complete recovery occurs.

In lawn-tennis, the right elbow is sometimes peculiarly

injured. This is now well recognised under the name of the "tennis-arm." It is due to injury of certain ligaments, or a small muscle near the elbow-joint. The only remedy is abstinence from the game for a prolonged period.

Football has the unenviable reputation of being the pastime which is, far above all others, liable to be accompanied by serious or even fatal accidents. Scarcely a week passes in the football season, but several accidents are recorded in the newspapers; and the following are but a few of many culled by the *Lancet* in the course of a few weeks:—"*A* had his right leg broken by a cross kick." "*B*, while engaged in a match, was kicked in the stomach; but, feeling better afterwards, he finished the game. He died, some time afterwards, from internal injuries." "*C* had his collar-bone broken." "*D's* left leg was broken clean through." "*E* received a severe kick on his left leg, by which two bones were broken just above the ankle." "*F*, while running with the ball, slipped forward and was fallen over by those pursuing him, his back being broken in the melée." Two cases have come under my own observation within the last month. In one, a knock on the chest by an opponent's knee caused complete collapse and unconsciousness, and the patient at the end of three weeks remains weak and shaken. In the other, the nose was cut across in a fall, and severe hæmorrhage occurred.

The Committee on Athletics at Harvard University, U.S.A., about a year ago, being convinced that the game of football, as at present played by college teams, is brutal and demoralising to players and spectators, and extremely dangerous, proposed to request the faculty to prohibit the game. We confess that this is, in our opinion, the only reasonable conclusion. Unless the game can be radically altered—for fatal accidents happen with both Rugby and Association play—the sooner another game takes its place the better. "Charging" should be forbidden; handling the ball and running with it should be forbidden; a hard and dangerous condition of the ground from frost should always be a sufficient reason for postponing the game; and the game should be confined entirely to the young, who seem to escape more readily than those of mature years. If, by some means, football could become true to its name, and not be foot-and-hand-ball, and if kicks could be made to fall more on the ball, and less on the shins and bodies of the players, its retention as a rational game might be tolerable.

The following notes are to accompany pages 133 and 134, which see:

NOTE I. — To free the lungs of water, protect the face while the body is gently turned face downwards; let some one stand astride the body, and joining his hands under the abdomen lift that part up high, making a few sharp jerks, the head hanging low, and the tongue drawn out. In a few moments, as soon as the water ceases to escape, turn the body over, and place a folded coat under the head and shoulders, so as to give firm support.

NOTE II. — Instant relief is often afforded by closing with firm pressure the free nostril, placing the mouth over the open mouth of the patient, and blowing forcibly.

INDEX.

	PAGE
Abrasions	136
Age in relation to school-work	71
Ague	4
Air, amount required	27
Air space in dormitories	93
Alternation of subjects	66
Arrangement of school-work	66
Artificial lighting	17
Astigmatism	110
Automatic flush-tanks	47, 53
Atrophy from disuse of organs	85
Back to seat	15
Bathing	102
Bites	135
Blackboard	16
Bleeding	136
Blood supply to brain	59
Books and eyesight	113
Boots	101
Boyle's mica-flap ventilator	34
Brain, structure and size	58
Brain-forcing	62
Bridgeport system of warming	44
Burns	137
Calisthenics	89
Central system of heating	41
Cesspools	52
Chicken-pox	119
Childhood, growth in	70
Chorea from school-work	64
Cleanliness	102
Cloak-rooms	10

	PAGE
Closed stoves	40
Closets	48
Closing schools for infectious disease	124
Clothing	99
Consumption from damp soil	4
Consumption from overcrowding	25
Consumption from overwork	68
Contusions	138
Corporal punishment	68
Corridors	10
Corsets	101
"Cram" system	65
Cubic space allowed	27
Damp clothing	100
Damp-proof course	7
Desks	12
Diet	94
Differentiation of functions of brain	59
Diphtheria	118
Direction of light	18
Disconnecting chamber	51
Dislocations	138
Distance and difference of desks	14
Dormitories	93
Drainage arrangements	46
Drain-pipe	51
Drainage of soil	4
Dress, in relation to food	99
Drowning	133
Dryness of air	26
Earth-closets	52

Index.

Early education, character of 61, 71
Effects of breathing impure air 24
Emulation, evils of, for girls 80
Epilepsy 132
Examinations . . . 67
Exercise 83
   ,, effects on brain, . 85
Extraction shafts for foul air 44
Eyeball, structure of, . . 104

Far-sightedness . . . 107
Fat, importance of, as food 96
Fits 130, 132
Floor and floor plan . . 9
Floor space per child. . 27
Food and work . . . 96
Football 139
Foreign bodies . . . 134
Foundation 7
Fractures 138
Furniture of school . . 12

Gas lights . . . 19
Gas stoves 39
German measles. . . 119
Glandular swellings . . 136
Ground-water . . . 3
Growth and development . 73
Growth, rate of . . 74, 78
Gymnastics 89

Hæmorrhage . . . 136
"Hardening" of children . 99
Headache, causes of . . 63
Height of children . 75, 78
Home lessons . . . 66
Hot air furnaces . . . 41
Hot water apparatus . . 42
Hypermetropia . . . 107
Hysteria 132

Incubation period . . 117
Infectious diseases . . 115
Infection, duration of . 120
Itch 127

Kindergarten system. . 61

Lawn-tennis arm . . 138
Lavatories 46
Liebreich on seat-backs . 15
Liebreich's chair. . . 86
Lighting of schools . . 17
Long sight 107

Measles 119
Mental exercise . . . 57
Merit grant 72
Mumps 120
Muscles, in relation to brain 60
Music exercises . . . 79
Muscular exercise . . 82
   ,, ,, effect on brain 84
Myopia 108

Natural ventilation . . 30
Needlework in relation to eyesight 114

Open fire-place . . . 37
Ophthalmia 129
Over-exertion, effects of . 85
Over-growth, dangers of . 74
Over-pressure . . . 65

Pan closet 48
Phthisis, see Consumption.
Physiology of respiration . 21
Pictures 16
Playgrounds . . . 6, 10
Posture, influence on health 12
Precocity 62
Puberty and school-work . 80
Punishments . . . 68

Quarantine period . . 122

Recreation 82
Recreative exercise . . 87
Rest 91
Ringworm 127
Rötheln 119
Rules respecting ventilation 30

Index. 143

	PAGE
Sanatorium	125
Scabies	127
Scald head	128
Scarlet fever	118
School-work after acute illness	64
School-work, duration of	72
Seats	13
Sensations in relation to brain	60
Sex in education	78, 80
Sheringham's valve ventilator	33
Short sight	108
Site of school	3
Sleep	92
Slope of desk	14
Smallpox	119
Soil, characters of	5
Soil-pipe	50
Sprains	138
Staircases	10
Steam,heating apparatus	42
Stings	135
St. Vitus's dance	130
Subsoil water	3
Suffocation	132
Surroundings of school	5
Swimming	103
Symptoms of onset of infectious disease	117

	PAGE
Temperature of air required	25
Tests for air impurities	23
Tobin's tubes	33
Training, effect on muscles, &c.	83
Tumbler and trough closets	49
Type of books	113
Urinals	47
Valveless closet	49
Ventilating closed stoves	40
" gas burners	16, 34
Ventilation	21
Walls, internal surface	8
" structure of	7
Warming, expense of	37
Water supply	97
Weighing students periodically	75
Weight of children	75, 78
Whooping cough	120
Window-area	18
Wounds	135
Writing lessons	113
Writing materials	114

SCIENCE.

Shaler's First Book in Geology.
For high school, or highest class in grammar school 1.00

Shaler's Teacher's Methods in Geology.
74 pages. An aid to the teacher using the above book 25

Shepard's Inorganic Chemistry.
Descriptive and Qualitative; experimental and inductive; leads the student to observe and think. For high schools and colleges 1.12

Shepard's Laboratory Note-Book.
Blanks for experiments; tables for the reaction of metallic salts, and pages for miscellaneous matter. Can be used with any chemistry 35

Chute's Practical Physics.
For high and preparatory schools studying physics experimentally. *In Press.*

Remsen's Organic Chemistry.
An Introduction to the study of the Compounds of Carbon. For all students of pure science, or of its application to the arts, medicine, etc. 1.20

Coit's Chemical Arithmetic.
With a short system of Elementary Qualitative Analysis. For high schools and colleges, .50

Grabfield and Burns' Chemical Problems.
For colleges, high and technical schools 50

Colton's Practical Zoölogy.
Gives a clear idea of the subject as a whole, by the careful study of a few typical animals, .80

William's Modern Petography.
An account of the application of the microscope to the study of geology . . .15

Clarke's Astronomical Lantern.
Intended to familiarize students with the constellations by comparing them with fac-similes on the lantern face. With seventeen slides 4.50

Clarke's How to Find the Stars.
Accompanies the above and helps to an acquaintance with the constellations . .15

Guides for Science-Teaching.
For instructing classes in Natural History in the lower grades.
No. 1. Hyatt's About Pebbles, .10. — No. 2. Goodale's A Few Common Plants, .15.— No. 3. Hyatt's Commercial and other Sponges, .20. — No. 4. Agassiz's First Lessons in Natural History, .20. — No. 5. Hyatt's Corals and Echinoderms, .25. — No. 6. Hyatt's Mollusca, .25. — No. 7. Hyatt's Worms and Crustacea, .25. — No. 12. Crosby's Common Minerals and Rocks, 40; cloth, .60. — No. 13. Richards' First Lessons in Minerals, .10. — No. 14. Bowditch's Physiology, .20. —. N.15. Clapp's Observation Lessons, .30

D. C. HEATH & CO., Boston, New York and Chicago.

BOOKS FOR TEACHERS.

Rousseau's Émile	$ .80
Pestalozzi's Leonard and Gertrude	.80
Richter's Levana: The Doctrine of Education,	1.25
Payne's Compayré's History of Pedagogy	1.60
Hall's Method of Teaching History	1.30
Gill's Systems of Education	1.00
Radestock's Habit in Education	.60
Rosmini's Method in Education	1.40
Peabody's Lectures to Kindergartners	1.00
Malleson's Early Training of Children	.60
Guides for Science Teaching, 10 to 40 cts. each.	
How to Use Wood-Working Tools	.50
Gustafson's Study of the Drink Question	1.60
Palmer's Temperance Teachings of Science	.50
Luce's Nature and Effects of Alcohol	.10
Teachers' Manual to Sheldon's History	.80
Teachers' Edition of Shaler's Geology	1.00
Badlam's Suggestive Lessons in Language and Reading	1.50
Williams's Modern Petrography	.25
Morris's Study of Latin in the Preparatory Course,	.25
Safford's Methods in Mathematical Teaching,	.25
Hall's How to Teach Reading and What to Read in School	.25
Genung's Study of Rhetoric in College Classes,	.25

IN PREPARATION.

Payne's Compayré's Lectures on Teaching.
De Garmo's Lindner's Man'l of Empirical Psychology.
MacAlister's Montaigne on Education.
Cox's Immanuel Kant on Pedagogy.
Woodward's Disciplinary Value of the Study of English.

D. C. HEATH & CO., Publishers, Boston, New York, and Chicago.

www.ingramcontent.com/pod-product-compliance
Lightning Source LLC
Chambersburg PA
CBHW030317170426
43202CB00009B/1043